CW00434110

Keynotes in medicine
for dental students

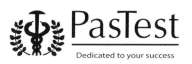

PasTest
Dedicated to your success

Keynotes in medicine for dental students

Douglas Hammond

BDS (Wales) MFGDP (UK) MBBS

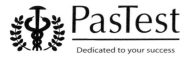

PasTest
Dedicated to your success

© 2008 PASTEST LTD
Egerton Court
Parkgate Estate
Knutsford
Cheshire
WA16 8DX

Telephone: 01565 752000

First Published 2008

ISBN: 1905635435

         9781905635436

A catalogue record for this book is available from the British Library.

The information contained within this book was obtained by the author from reliable sources. However, while every effort has been made to ensure its accuracy, no responsibility for loss, damage or injury occasioned to any person acting or refraining from action as a result of information contained herein can be accepted by the publishers or author.

PasTest Revision Books and Intensive Courses

PasTest has been established in the field of postgraduate medical education since 1972, providing revision books and intensive study courses for doctors preparing for their professional examinations.

Books and courses are available for the following specialties:

MRCGP, MRCP Parts 1 and 2, MRCPCH Parts 1 and 2, MRCS, MRCOG Parts 1 and 2, DRCOG, DCH, FRCA, Dentistry.

For further details contact:
PasTest, Freepost, Knutsford, Cheshire WA16 7BR
Tel: 01565 752000   Fax: 01565 650264
www.pastest.co.uk   enquiries@pastest.co.uk

Front cover image ©TEK IMAGE/SCIENCE PHOTO LIBRARY

Text prepared by Carnegie Book Production, Lancaster

Printed and bound in the UK by CPI Antony Rowe

Contents

About the Author   vii

Foreword   viii

Introduction   ix

1. Introduction to History Taking and Clinical Examination   1

2. Atheroma and Coronary Artery Disease   7

3. Cardiac Valves and Bacterial Endocarditis   19

4. Heart Failure and Hypertension   27

5. Deep Vein Thrombosis, Pulmonary Embolism and
Cardiac Arrhythmias   33

6. Airway Disorders   41

7. Chest Infections and Lung Cancer   49

8. Tubular Gut   55

9. Liver and Pancreatic Disease   61

10. Diabetes Mellitus   69

11. Pituitary Gland and Gonads   77

12. Thyroid and Adrenals   83

13. Bone Disease and Parathyroids   91

14. Arthritis and Connective Tissue Disease   99

15. Renal Disease   105

16. Anaemia and Bleeding Disorders   111

17. Headache and Cranial Nerve Defects   119

18. Loss of Consciousness, Fits and Coma   129

19. Neurological Disorders   133

20. Psychiatry for Dental Students   139

21. Childhood Illnesses   145

22. Dermatology   153

23. Oral Manifestations of Medical Conditions   159

24. Sexually Transmitted Diseases and AIDS   163

25. Clinical Genetics   169

26. Examination of the Acutely Unwell Patient   173

Index   177

About the Author

**Douglas Hammond BDS (Wales) MFGDP (UK) MBBS
(UCL and Royal Free Medical School)**
Academic F2 doctor in Maxillofacial Surgery

Douglas graduated from Cardiff Dental Hospital and completed various hospital and practice jobs. He then began working as a part-time lecturer in Oral and Maxillofacial Surgery at the Royal London Hospital in 2002, whilst embarking on a medicine degree at University College London. He completed his medicine degree in June 2007, and passed MRCS part A at the first sitting. He is completing his Foundation training and from there he hopes to continue into specialist training in Oral and Maxillofacial Surgery. Douglas has recently been appointed honorary lecturer at the Royal College of Surgeons.

Foreword

As stated in the GDC review of curricula by a framework document 'The First Five Years', human disease education in relation to dentistry remains a key area in the education of dental students. The importance of a book such as this, in learning and acquiring these essential professional skills, cannot be underestimated.

As you progress through your dental career, understanding the basis of medical problems becomes vital in improving your ability to manage patients and plays a key role in prevention of chronic medical diseases. As medical science is fast progressing, it is important to regularly update your knowledge and this book provides a helpful reference for qualified dentists needing to 'polish' their skills.

The author of this text has given us a fresh perspective on medicine in relation to dentistry. It is a well-written, concise and helpful book which I am sure will become a main 'staple' text for all dentists and members of the dental team.

Tara Renton
Professor in Oral Surgery
Kings College London Dental Institute of Psychiatry, KCL

Introduction

This book will provide both the dental undergraduate and singly qualified maxillofacial SHO with a concise and helpful guide to the basics of medicine. Presenting the essential knowledge base for your needs in both dental practice and also in a hospital-based setting, it covers most of the common conditions, management and treatment which you will come across. The book also covers the curriculum for the dental undergraduate medicine stem and also for the new MJDF exam.

Douglas Hammond

1

Introduction to History Taking and Clinical Examination

Dental students should already be familiar with the concept of history taking and physical examination of patients. In clinical medicine, the history must encompass a greater variety of systems, in comparison to a dental history, and is followed by a complete physical examination. A number of points should be borne in mind:

1. The history is vital and will often lead you to the diagnosis. If you have no idea of the diagnosis after taking the history, do not expect the examination to help you much either.
2. Allow the patient to speak.
3. Learn to listen.
4. Avoid leading questions.

A medical history usually follows a standard format. To look professional and make a good impression, always start with the following information: name of the patient, age, ethnicity, marital status and occupation. Then move on to the history.

Presenting complaint

The presenting complaint is best recorded in the patient's own words rather than as your interpretation.

History of presenting complaint

Especially for pain, it is useful to follow the mnemonic *SOCRATES*. This stands for:

S ite

O nset

C haracter

R adiation

A ssociated symptoms

T emporal – when does it hurt. morning/evening, constant, occasionally, etc.

E xacerbating or relieving factors

S everity – ask the patient to rate the pain on a scale of between 0 and 10, where 10 is the worst pain imaginable.

Relevant medical history

The medical history is vital. Ask especially about any visits to a general practitioner (GP) or a hospital in the past 2 years and the diagnosis that was made. Ask about diabetes, hypertension, angina and heart attacks, valve problems or rheumatic fever, infectious diseases and bleeding problems. A good list of items to run through is:

- any serious illnesses
- heart or chest trouble
- heart attack (*it should be myocardial infarction, but patients understand this better*) or stroke
- rheumatic fever
- bronchitis
- diabetes
- asthma
- hay fever
- eczema
- hepatitis
- bleeding problems
- epilepsy
- tuberculosis
- admissions to hospital
- operations
- could you be pregnant
- any recent visits to your GP.

Family history

You should always ask about parents and siblings: whether they are alive and well, or if they are dead, then what did they die of and at what age. You should also ask if there are any hereditary conditions or cancers which family members may have had. Also ask about heart disease and diabetes, as these conditions have strong familial trends.

Drug history

You should ask whether the patient is taking any medications, which ones they have been taking recently, and whether they have any allergies. Always make a very clear note of steroid use and allergies.

Social history

This should include:

- smoking history
- alcohol intake
- use of recreational drugs
- their job
- stress – ask the patient if there are any new problems in their life, as a way of enquiring about stress.
- marital status
- whether they have any children.

Systems enquiry

This is a series of questions aimed at uncovering any symptoms in other systems which the patient have not volunteered themselves. The questions are asked as direct questions requiring direct answers. Positive answers should lead to further questions aimed at fully documenting the symptoms. The key symptoms you should ask about are:

- *Cardiovascular system* (CVS): chest pain, shortness of breath at rest and during exercise, angina, palpitations, ankle swelling, intermittent claudication, nocturnal dyspnoea.
- *Respiratory system*: shortness of breath, wheeze, cough, sputum, haemoptysis, paroxysmal nocturnal dyspnoea and orthopnoea.
- *Gastrointestinal system*: appetite, weight, dysphagia, indigestion, vomiting, haematemesis, abdominal pain, bowels, bleeding per rectum.
- *Neurological system*: fits, faints, headache, diplopia, paraesthesia/ anaesthesia, muscle weakness, eyesight, memory.
- *Musculoskeletal system*: joint pains, stiffness, skin rashes.
- *Urogenital system*: nocturia, polyuria, dysuria, haematuria, prostatism, period cycle, dysmenorrhoea, amenorrhoea, discharge, impotence.

Physical examination

As a dentist you are unlikely ever to perform a full medical examination, unless you are working in the maxillofacial surgery unit in a hospital. However, you should be able to recognise common physical findings such as rheumatoid hands, skin rashes and thyroid enlargement. You should also be able to recognise signs of heart failure and respiratory distress. The technique of physical examination will be demonstrated to you at one of the clinical sessions. Important physical signs you should be able to recognise will be highlighted throughout the course. Physical examination is performed in a specific order:

1. Always take the history first
2. Inspection
3. Palpation
4. Percussion
5. Auscultation.

2

Atheroma and Coronary Artery Disease

Normal anatomy and physiology

The prime function of the heart is to pump blood around the body. Cardiac muscle (ie the myocardium) contracts powerfully in response to physiological demands. Starling's curve defines the relationship between the stretch on the myocardium and the force of contraction. The rate of contraction (ie the heart rate) is determined by a physiological pacemaker in the right atrium (the sino-atrial node). Essentially, if the heart is working harder it requires a greater supply of blood.

The myocardium is too thick and metabolically active to obtain sufficient oxygen and nutrient supply from the blood within the ventricles and is supplied by the coronary arteries. Both the left and right coronary arteries arise from the aorta. The left coronary artery divides into the left anterior descending and the left circumflex arteries; together with the right coronary artery these are often referred to as the 'three coronary arteries'.

Blood flow to the myocardium is greatest during diastole. In systole, the myocardium contracts and this impedes blood flow through the coronary arteries. With increasing heart rate, the diastolic interval shortens since systole is always of a finite length. Thus coronary blood flow is particularly increased during tachycardia.

Atherosclerosis

Atherosclerosis is the process by which the arteries become narrower, hence impeding blood flow. Flow through a blood vessel is related to the square of the diameter, so even small amounts of narrowing lead to relatively large decreases in blood flow. Atherosclerosis occurs as part of ageing, but it is more prevalent in Western societies. The first changes that are seen are slightly raised 'fatty streaks' in the aorta in teenage. With increasing age, the streaks enlarge to form atheromatous plaques. The plaques are rich in lipid and also contain cells such as fibroblasts and macrophages. As the plaques enlarge, they slowly encroach on the diameter of the vessel. If the endothelial covering of the plaque breaks down (fissuring), a thrombus can form on the plaque, leading to rapid occlusion of the vessel. Risk factors for atheroma formation include:

- hypertension
- high lipid (cholesterol/triglycerides) states
- positive family history
- men
- diabetes
- smokers.

Symptoms

Much of an atheroma is laid down silently. When one or more of the coronary arteries is sufficiently narrowed, blood flow to the myocardium is limited. Initially symptoms will only come on with exercise. The increased heart rate and increased power of contraction demands more blood, which cannot flow through the narrow artery. This leads to the build up of lactic acid in the muscle and stimulation of pain fibres, leading to angina. Taking a history is very relevant when angina is suspected. If the pain is relieved by leaning forward, the diagnosis of pericarditis is more likely. If the pain is relieved by taking antacids, a diagnosis of gastro-oesophageal reflux disease is more likely.

Angina pectoris literally means pain in the chest or throat. The pain can be difficult to distinguish from other causes of chest pain but the classical description is of dull, pressing pain in the centre of the chest. Patients may describe it as a weight on their chest that may radiate to the left arm, both arms or the right arm, throat or neck. It may be present only in the jaw. Classically the pain is relieved promptly by rest and is predictable, ie the same level of exertion tends to bring on the pain. When the atheroma is severe, or if the plaque has fissured, a patient may develop increasing pain with lesser exertion, or even pain at rest. This is termed **unstable angina**. It warns that a myocardial infarct may be imminent, and is a medical emergency.

Treatment of angina

- Lifestyle changes: encourage the patient to stop smoking, to exercise and try to lose weight.
- Modification of risk factors: hypertension, diabetes, etc.
- Aspirin (75–150 mg) – reduces risk of mortality by 34%.
- Beta blockers, eg atenolol 50–100 mg/day. These drugs slow the heart and reduce the force of contraction, unless contraindicated (asthma, chronic obstructive pulmonary disease, left ventricular failure, bradycardia).

- Calcium antagonists – amlodipine 5 mg/day. This reduces the heart rate and force of contraction and dilates arterioles.
- Nitrates (eg glyceryl trinitrate (GTN)) – venodilators for relief of symptoms, given as GTN spray or sublingual tablets. If used as prophylaxis, longer-acting nitrates, eg isosorbide mononitrate 10–30 mg, should be given, however, these are not well tolerated as they lead to headaches.
- Statins – check if total cholesterol is > 4 mmol/l and treat with a statin. Statins are HMG co-A reductase inhibitors and reduce the patient's low-density lipoprotein (LDL) cholesterol level. Patients taking statins require liver function monitoring, and occasionally a patient will develop the serious side effect of myositis.

Unstable angina is treated with bed rest, intravenous nitrates and heparin.

Further investigations

Exercise testing

Exercise testing defines the severity of symptoms. Electrocardiographic (ECG) changes (usually ST depression) after low workload suggests the need for further intervention. It is also used after patients have had a myocardial infarction to assess recovery. Exercise testing is sometimes used in patients with atypical chest pain and may be helpful in some patients with asymptomatic coronary artery disease. It has a role in patients with asymptomatic angina or those with chest pain when diagnosis is in doubt.

Angiography

In this test, a catheter is passed into the femoral or brachial artery and fed through the diseased coronary artery. A dye is injected and serial X-rays taken. The degree of narrowing can be seen on the radiographs.

Coronary artery bypass grafting (CABG)

In this procedure, narrowed arteries are bypassed with grafts taken from veins from the leg or internal mammary artery.

Angioplasty

In this technique, a balloon in fed into the narrowed artery and blown up to make the diameter larger. Restenosis after the procedure may be problematical.

Myocardial infarction and acute coronary syndromes

Acute coronary syndromes (ACS) include unstable angina and evolving myocardial infarction, which share a common underlying pathology – plaque rupture, thrombosis and inflammation. However, rarely, ACS may arise because of emboli or coronary spasm in normal arteries. This means that ACS can be divided into ACS with ST elevation and ACS without ST elevation.

Myocardial infarction is defined as when the blood supply to a part of the heart is suddenly interrupted and becomes insufficient to maintain myocardial viability. The most common cause is thrombosis of an atheromatous plaque. Such plaques need not be particularly large and there may not have been any angina before the event. Symptoms can vary:

- Sudden loss of consciousness and/or death: this is because of the heart beating irregularly (usually ventricular fibrillation), so that no blood is pumped to the brain.
- Severe chest pain lasting for more than 20 minutes: worse than angina, often described as crushing. It is associated with nausea, vomiting and sweating patient looks 'grey'.
- Shortness of breath: due to acute left ventricular failure – the heart cannot pump blood away from the lungs, which fill with fluid.
- Palpitations: due to the heart beating irregularly (arrhythmia).

Investigations

ECGs are performed to demonstrate a number of important features.

- Classical changes occur when the heart muscle is dying (ST elevation). Depending on which ECG leads are affected, the right or left coronary artery can be implicated.
- Heart rate and rhythm can be checked.
- Evidence of previous infarcts or hypertension may be present.

The ECG in Figure 2.1 shows ST elevation in anterior leads V1–V6 and in leads I and aVL. This indicates an anterolateral myocardial infarction.

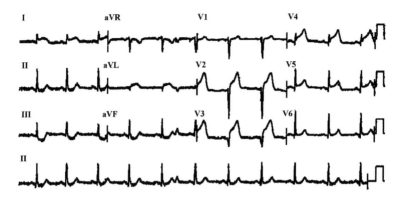

Figure 2.1 An ECG.

A chest radiograph (CXR) will show any fluid in the lungs (pulmonary oedema).

Troponin levels

Troponin is an enzyme. It is released from dying heart muscle and if measured in serial blood samples starting 12 hours after the onset of chest pain it helps make the diagnosis of a heart attack. If a troponin I level is greater than 0.15 12 hours after the onset of pain, it may signify a myocardial infarction.

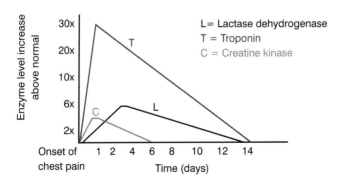

Figure 2.2 Cardiac enzyme changes in myocardial infarction.

Management of acute myocardial infarction

The mnemonic *MONA* is important for remembering the management of patients whom you suspect are having an acute myocardial infarction. It stands for:

Morphine – 5–10 mg iv + an anti-emetic, eg metoclopramide 10 mg iv
Oxygen – high flow oxygen via face mask
N itrates – GTN sublingually
A spirin – 300 mg (chewed).

After the above initial management, the next part is controversial and depends on each hospital's policy. Some hospitals prefer thrombolysis and other hospitals prefer primary angioplasty.

Thrombolytics, eg streptokinase and alteplase – are drugs given iv, which help dissolve blood clots, limiting the size of infarct and hence improving outcome. The sooner thrombolytics are administered, the better.

Indications
- ST elevation of > 2 mm in two or more chest leads
- ST elevation of > 1 mm in two or more limb leads.

Contraindications
- Recent surgery (< 2 weeks)
- Internal bleeding
- Traumatic cardiopulmonary resuscitation (CPR)
- Liver disease
- Oesophageal varices
- Recent haemorrhagic stroke
- Suspected aortic dissection.

Emergency angiogram/angioplasty

This is beginning to be favoured in more hospitals, as the evidence for thrombolysis has been decreasing.

Subsequent management after angioplasty or thrombolysis

- Bed rest for 48 hours with continuous ECG monitoring.
- Daily 12-lead ECG, urea and electrolytes (U&E), troponin measurements for 3 days.
- Prophylaxis against thromboembolism, eg heparin 5000 U/12 h subcutaneously, until mobile. Consider warfarin anticoagulation for 3 months. Continue low dose aspirin (75–150 mg) daily, indefinitely. Aspirin reduces vascular events by 29%.
- Start a β blocker, eg metoprolol 50 mg four times daily to decrease the pulse rate to less than 60 bpm; continue for at least a year. Beta blockers reduce mortality by 25% in those who have had a previous myocardial infarction.
- Consider angiotensin-converting enzyme (ACE) inhibitors in all patients. ACE inhibitors reduce mortality by 25–30% in a 2-year period in those with evidence of heart failure.
- Start a statin. Cholesterol reduction post-myocardial infarction has been shown to have benefits in those with normal and raised cholesterol levels.
- Address modifiable risk factors, eg smoking, diet. Identify and treat diabetes mellitus and hypertension.

Other atheromatous diseases

Atheroma may affect the carotid or cerebral arteries, predisposing to strokes. Narrowing of the renal arteries may result in hypertension and renal impairment. Aneurysms in large arteries (eg abdominal aorta) result because the atheromatous process weakens the vessel wall. Peripheral vascular disease is the term given to ischaemic symptoms in the limbs – in severe cases, there is intermittent claudication, ulceration and eventually gangrene requiring amputation.

Cardiovascular examination

1. **WIPER**: Wash hands, Introduce, Permission, Expose (remove clothing required), Reposition.
2. **Observe**: look at the patient and their surroundings, for example, does the patient have a walking stick? Do they have an oxygen tank nearby? Do they have inhalers or their ETN spray to hand? A great deal can be learnt by just watching the patient.

3. **Hands**: check the temperature of the hands and perfusion, look for clubbing of the fingers, petechiae and splinter haemorrhages.
   - Clubbing
   - Splinter haemorrhages

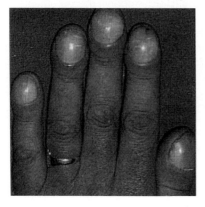

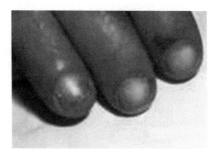

Figure 2.4 Splinter haemorrhages.

Figure 2.3 Finger clubbing.

4. **Pulse**: check the pulse. Comment on its rate, regularity and volume.
5. **Blood pressure**: offer to take it.
6. **Face**: check the conjunctiva for anaemia and jaundice, look for xanthelasma, and look intraorally for central cyanosis.
7. **Neck**: check the carotid pulse and the jugular venous pressure (JVP).
8. **Chest**: stop and observe the chest again. Look for any asymmetry or scars. Feels for the apex beat of the heart. This should be in the fifth intercostal space, in the mid-clavicular line. Feel for any heaves or thrills.
9. **Auscultate**: remember the mnemonic (**A P**lace **T**o **M**eet).
   - aortic valve (second intercostal space, right sternal edge)
   - pulmonary valve (second intercostal space, left sternal edge)
   - tricuspid valve (left lower sternal edge)
   - mitral valve (apex of heart, to be listened with the bell of the stethoscope).

In addition:

   - listen to the carotids for bruits
   - listen to the bases of the lungs for crackles and wheezes.

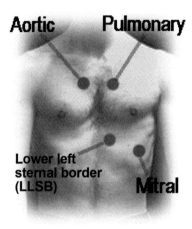

Figure 2.5 Auscultation sites.

10. **Also**: look for oedema and feel for an abdominal aortic aneurysm.
11. **Pulses**: feel the femoral, popliteal, posterior tibial and dorsalis pedis pulses.

Example ECGs

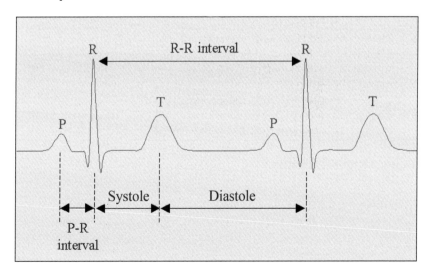

Figure 2.6 Normal ECG.

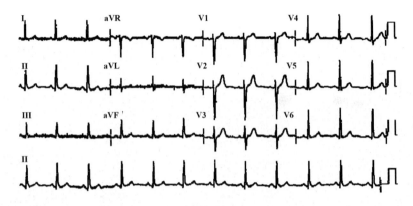

Figure 2.7 No P wave, and irregularly irregular rhythm.

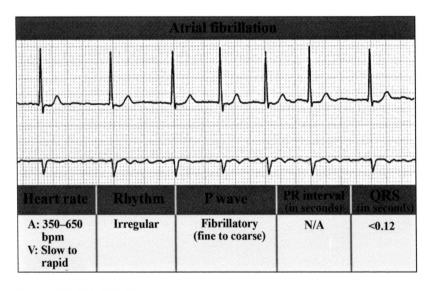

Heart rate	Rhythm	P wave	PR interval (in seconds)	QRS (in seconds)
A: 350–650 bpm V: Slow to rapid	Irregular	Fibrillatory (fine to coarse)	N/A	<0.12

Figure 2.8 Atrial fibrillation.

3
Cardiac Valves and Bacterial Endocarditis

Normal anatomy and physiology

The right side of the heart receives systemic venous return and pumps it to the lungs for gaseous exchange. The left side of the heart pumps oxygenated blood to the periphery. The main pumping chambers are the ventricles, and the atria act as 'pump primers'. The four cardiac valves prevent backflow of blood:

- tricuspid valve: between the right atrium and right ventricle
- pulmonary valve: between the right ventricle and pulmonary artery
- mitral valve: between the left atrium and left ventricle
- aortic valve: between the left ventricle and aorta.

During systole, the tricuspid and mitral valves shut and the pulmonary and aortic valves open. During diastole, the tricuspid and mitral valves are open and the pulmonary and aortic valves are shut. The valves are held in place by fibrous rings. The papillary muscles holding the mitral valve are important as they can be damaged by myocardial infarction. Blood flow through a normal valve is usually silent.

The first heart sound corresponds to closure of the tricuspid and mitral valves. The second heart sound is due to closure of the pulmonary and aortic valves. The interval between the first and second heart sounds is systole and should be silent. The interval between the second and first heart sound is diastole and also should be silent.

Heart murmurs

When thinking about a murmur, consider it in terms of its character, timing, loudness, area where it is the loudest, radiation and accentuating manoeuvres.

Murmurs are heard when a valve is roughened or narrow (stenosis), or if a valve is leaky (regurgitant) (Figure 3.1).

- If the aortic or pulmonary valves are stenotic, an ejection systolic (harsh) murmur results.
- If the aortic or pulmonary valves are leaky, an early diastolic (blowing) murmur results.
- If the mitral or tricuspid valves are stenotic, a diastolic (low pitched) murmur results.

- If the mitral or tricuspid valves are leaky, a pan-systolic (harsh) murmur results.
- Aortic stenosis murmurs tend to radiate to the neck.
- Mitral stenosis murmurs tend to radiate to the axilla.
- Very loud murmurs may be accompanied by a palpable 'thrill'.

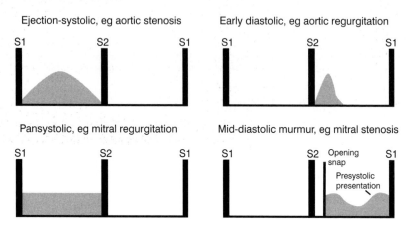

Figure 3.1 Heart sounds and murmurs.

S1 is the sound of the tricuspid and mitral valve closing, and S2 is the sound of the aortic and pulmonary valves closing.

- Aortic stenosis is a narrowing of the aortic valve so this occurs in systole (between S1 and S2).
- Mitral regurgitation is incompetence of the mitral valve. This means that blood is leaking through the valve during systole, therefore the murmur occurs in systole (between S1 and S2).
- Aortic regurgitation is incompetence of the aortic valve. This means that blood is leaking through the valve during systole, therefore the murmur occurs in systole (between S2 and S1).
- Mitral stenosis is a narrowing of the mitral valve so this occurs in systole (between S2 and S1).

Symptoms and signs

These depend on which valve is affected, and this can generally be deduced from a knowledge of cardiac physiology. Thus, aortic stenosis will cause low pulse pressure, left ventricular hypertrophy and eventually signs of left heart failure. Mitral stenosis causes right atrial enlargement and pulmonary hypertension.

Causes of valvular heart disease

- Congenital, eg congenitally bicuspid aortic valve; Marfan's syndrome
- Ischaemia, eg papillary muscle infarction
- Dysfunction, eg dilation of mitral valve ring in heart failure
- Bacterial endocarditis: acute, subacute.

Investigation of heart murmurs

- CXR may show classical features of valve disease.
- Echocardiogram allows valve to be 'visualised' and gradients calculated.

Rheumatic fever

Rheumatic fever is no longer a common disease in Western countries, however, it is still common in the developing world. The effects of previous infection are still commonly seen in the UK. Peak incidence is in the 5–15 year age range. The disease is a sequel of acute infection with Lancefield group A β-haemolytic streptococcus, which triggers rheumatic fever 2–4 weeks later in susceptible individuals. The most common initial infection is sore throat, which may be trivial. An antibody to the carbohydrate cell wall of the streptococcus cross-reacts with the valve tissue and may cause permanent damage to the valves.

Diagnosis

Diagnosis is based on the revised Jones's criteria. There must be evidence of recent streptococcal infection plus presence of two major criteria, or one major plus two minor criteria.

- Evidence of streptococcal infection:
    - recent streptococcal infection
    - history of scarlet fever
    - positive throat swab
    - anti-streptolysin O titre (ASO) titre > 200 U/ml.
- Major criteria
    - carditis
    - arthritis: a flitting polyarthritis affects 70% of those with rheumatic fever
    - subcutaneous nodules: small mobile and painless nodules on extensor surfaces and the spine

- erythema marginatum: geographical-type rash with red border and clear centre on the trunk
- Sydenham's chorea: also known as St Vitus dance – causes involuntary movements.
- Minor criteria
  - fever
  - raised C-reactive protein (CRP) level
  - arthralgia
  - previous rheumatic fever
  - prolonged P-R interval.

Management

- Bed rest
- Benzylpenicillin
- Aspirin.

Prognosis

Sixty per cent of patients with carditis will develop chronic rheumatic heart disease:

- mitral valve – 70%
- aortic valve – 40%
- tricuspid – 10%
- pulmonary – 2%.

Valves affected by previous rheumatic fever are at risk of bacterial endocarditis.

Infective endocarditis

Remember: fever + new murmur = endocarditis until proved otherwise.

Fifty per cent of all endocarditis occurs on previously normal valves. It follows an acute course and presents with acute heart failure. Endocarditis on abnormal valves tends to run a subacute course. Predisposing cardiac lesions are: aortic or mitral valve disease; tricuspid valves in iv drug users; prosthetic heart valves; coarctation; and ventricular septal defects.

Causes

The disease is due to infection of a valve following transient bacteriaemia, eg dental work, catheterisation, cannulation, or surgery. Quite often no precipitating cause can be demonstrated. Common causative organisms are *Streptococcus viridans* (35–50% of all cases), *Streptococcus faecalis* and *Staphylococcus aureus*. Right-sided valves are infected in iv drug users. Infected 'vegetations' form on the heart valves which may erode and lead to acute heart failure. The vegetations may embolise, causing strokes.

Symptoms and signs

- Fever
- Weight loss
- Malaise
- Night sweats
- Finger clubbing
- Splenomegaly
- Anaemia
- Mycotic aneurysms
- Splinter haemorrhages
- Roth spots
- Osler's nodes
- Changing heart murmurs
- Heart failure if valve ruptures
- Stroke if mycotic aneurysm bursts.

Investigations

- Full blood count (FBC) + Erythrocyte sedimentation rate (ESR)
- Blood cultures
- Echocardiography
- CXR
- Mid-stream urine (MSU) for haematuria

Diagnosis

Duke's criteria: two major or one major and three minor or all five minor criteria for a positive diagnosis.

- Major criteria:
    - positive blood culture
    - endocardium involved (positive echocardiogram or new valvular regurgitation).

- Minor criteria:
    - predisposition, eg cardiac lesion; iv drug use
    - fever > 38° Celsius
    - vascular/immunological signs
    - positive blood culture that does not meet major criteria
    - positive echocardiogram that does not meet major criteria.

Management

- Antibiotics: benzylpenicillin; gentamicin; flucloxacillin.
- Antibiotic prophylaxis for subacute endocarditis.
- Amoxicillin 3 g orally 1 h pre-operatively (can give a further 3 g 6 h later)
- High-risk patients sometimes also receive gentamicin 80–120 mg (remember – renal function).
- Patients allergic to penicillin may be given clindamycin, teicoplanin or vancomycin.

Antibiotic prophylaxis is a controversial area, and the guidance changes frequently. Dentists should consult the current copy of the *British National Formulary* (*BNF*) for up-to-date guidelines.

Congenital heart disease

A variety of congenital cardiac abnormalities may occur. They are broadly divided into cyanotic forms (shunt blood left to right) and acyanotic forms. Acyanotic forms may become cyanotic with shunt reversal (due to development of pulmonary hypertension). Patients are at risk of infective endocarditis and require prophylactic antibiotics, prior to dental treatment.

4
Heart Failure and Hypertension

Normal physiology

The left ventricle pumps blood efficiently through the aortic valve during systole. The pulse wave may be checked at superficial arteries. The systolic blood pressure is the pressure generated in the arteries by the action of the heart. It is normally enough to allow adequate perfusion of all tissues. Organs in special need of adequate perfusion include the brain and the kidneys. During diastole, the aortic valve is closed, preventing backflow of blood into the left ventricle. The diastolic pressure is a measure of the resistance to blood flow in the arterial circulation. The pulse pressure is the difference between the systolic and diastolic pressures.

The venous blood returns to the right atrium and then into the right ventricle. During systole, blood is pumped through the pulmonary valve into the pulmonary artery and thus into the lungs for oxygenation. The blood returns via the pulmonary veins into the left atrium.

Heart failure

Heart failure usually implies impaired pump action by the heart; this may be due to diseases of the myocardium or valves.

Causes

- Ischaemic heart disease, eg previous myocardial infarction
- Arrhythmias
- Valvular heart disease
- Cardiomyopathies
- Myocarditis
- High-output states, eg thyrotoxicosis, anaemia.

Left ventricular failure

Left ventricular failure results in raised pulmonary venous pressure and causes leakage of plasma into the alveoli (pulmonary oedema). It presents with shortness of breath, paroxysmal nocturnal dyspnoea (can also occur in asthma) and orthopnoea. In severe cases, patients will cough up pink, frothy sputum. Patients may be cyanosed and tachycardic with low systemic blood pressure and crackles at the bases of the lungs and have signs of pleural effusion. A CXR shows alveolar fluid with enlarged pulmonary vasculature (upper lobe diversion). Echocardiogram shows poorly functioning left ventricle.

Right ventricular failure

Right ventricular failure results in raised peripheral venous pressure causing peripheral oedema (pitting). The liver becomes congested and this may be palpable on examination. Oedema of the gut wall prevents adequate absorption of drugs and nutrients. The jugular venous pressure may be visibly raised in the neck.

Treatment

- Correct any remediable cause, eg arrhythmia, anaemia, ischaemia
- Stop negatively inotropic or chronotropic drugs
- Diuretics
- ACE inhibitors
- Fluid restriction
- Bed rest
- Oxygen
- Heart transplantation.

Hypertension

There is a continuous distribution of systolic and diastolic blood pressures in the general population. Epidemiological studies have shown that raised diastolic blood pressure (> 90 mmHg) and raised systolic blood pressure (> 150 mmHg) are associated with an increased risk of death from strokes and myocardial infarction. The lower the blood pressure, the lower the risk. Ninety-five per cent of hypertension is essential (ie no cause is found). Secondary hypertension may occur in:

- pregnancy (associated with proteinuria and oedema in pre-eclampsia)
- renal disease
- endocrine disease (eg Cushing's syndrome, acromegaly, Conn's syndrome, phaeochromocytoma)
- coarctation of the aorta.

Blood pressure should be carefully measured in the rested, supine patient. Consistently elevated pressures almost always require treatment.

Treatment

- Lifestyle changes
- Losing weight
- Diuretics
- ACE inhibitors
- Beta blockers
- Calcium antagonists
- Other drugs such as venodilators.

Beware of stopping anti-hypertensives suddenly, especially β blockers.

Episodes of light-headedness or falls in elderly patients may suggest over-treatment with anti-hypertensives. In this situation, it is important to measure the blood pressure when the patient is both lying and standing.

Symptoms

There are usually no symptoms. Some patients do complain of headaches and nose bleeds but this may be a spurious association.

Signs

- Forceful cardiac impulse
- Hypertensive retinopathy
- Signs of renal failure (cause or effect of hypertension).

Malignant (accelerated) hypertension

- This is a rapid rise in blood pressure.
- May be associated with rapid deterioration of renal function or encephalopathy.

5

Deep Vein Thrombosis, Pulmonary Embolism and Cardiac Arrhythmias

Deep vein thrombosis

Venous blood normally returns promptly to the right atrium via the large veins. The passage of blood from the lower limbs up to the heart is aided by the presence of valves within the veins (to prevent backflow) and the pumping action of contracting muscles in close proximity to the veins. Obesity, immobility or damage to the wall of the vein may impair venous return. Sluggish blood in the venous circulation may produce a thrombus.

- Clot: coagulation of blood outside the body or after death.
- Thrombus: coagulation of blood in vivo.
- Embolus: fragment of thrombus which becomes dislodged.

Thrombosis is enhanced by Virchow's triad:

- stasis
- hypercoagulability
- damage to vessel wall.

All these factors are commonly present after surgery and in patients who are ill for other reasons, eg heart failure. Deep vein thrombosis (DVT) usually occurs in the lower limbs. It may be symptomatic or present as a swollen and painful leg. The differential diagnosis includes cellulitis or a ruptured Baker's cyst. Clinically it can be very difficult to be certain if a DVT is present – Doppler studies and venograms aid the diagnosis.

The most important consequence of a DVT is pulmonary embolism. Therefore all patients with DVT must be admitted to hospital. Treatment is with anticoagulation – initially iv (or subcutaneous (sc)) heparin. Heparin has a rapid onset of action and helps lyse the thrombus. Subsequently, anticoagulation is continued with oral warfarin for at least 3 months. Patients may be left with a chronically swollen leg (post-phlebitic syndrome).

The risk of DVT may be lessened by encouraging early mobilisation after surgery, and with the prophylactic administration of daily enoxaparin. Patients should stop smoking and lose weight. The contraceptive pill is a risk factor and women should consider stopping the pill prior to surgery. Graduated stockings may reduce the incidence of DVT if worn correctly.

Pulmonary embolus

This occurs when a fragment of a deep vein thrombus dislodges and passes through the right side of the heart and into the pulmonary circulation. Other rarer causes include air, bone (following fracture), amniotic fluid (following labour), tumour or embolus from right-sided bacterial endocarditis.

A massive pulmonary embolus may lodge at the bifurcation of the pulmonary arteries and totally block right-sided cardiac output. This results in sudden collapse and death. Cardiopulmonary resuscitation may revive the patient if the chest massage can break down the embolus so that it passes more distally into the pulmonary circulation.

A large pulmonary embolus presents as pleuritic chest pain, sudden shortness of breath, cough, haemoptysis (bright red), tachypnoea, tachycardia, atrial fibrillation, raised jugular venous pressure, pleural rub and perhaps signs of the underlying DVT.

Small pulmonary emboli may present as just mild shortness of breath or pleuritic chest pain. Recurrent small pulmonary emboli may be silent and only present as established chronic pulmonary hypertension and right heart failure.

Risk factors

Risk factors for deep vein thrombosis pulmonary embolism include any cause of immobility or hypercoagulability:

- recent surgery
- recent stroke or myocardial infarction
- malignancy
- thrombophilia
- prolonged bed rest
- pregnancy
- use of contraceptive pill
- smoking.

Investigations

- Chest radiograph – may be normal but may show linear atelectasis or pleural effusion.

- ECG – normal or sinus tachycardia, signs of right heart strain. Academics talk about S1Q3T3 pattern, but this is rarely seen.
- D-dimer test – blood tests are sensitive but not specific for DVT.
- Arterial gases – typically show hypoxaemia and hypocapnia.
- Computed tomography (CT) pulmonary angiogram – may visualise the embolus.
- Echocardiogram – shows right ventricular failure. Chronic cases show right ventricular hypertrophy and may indicate pulmonary hypertension.
- Life-threatening pulmonary emboli may be treated surgically (embolectomy) or by the infusion of thrombolytics such as tissue plasminogen activator (tPA) or streptokinase.
- Other pulmonary emboli are treated with heparin and then warfarin. Patients with recurrent pulmonary emboli are prescribed warfarin lifelong.

Cardiac arrhythmias

Normally the heart rate and rhythm are generated in the sino-atrial node – hence sinus rhythm.

- The atrium may fire off extra beats – atrial ectopics.
- The atrium may fire off completely randomly – atrial fibrillation (AF).
- The atrium may fire off very quickly but regularly – supraventricular tachycardia (SVT).

Atrial electrical activity is passed to the ventricles through the atrio-ventricular node.

- The ventricle may fire spontaneously – ventricular ectopics (VEs).
- The ventricle may fire spontaneously, rapidly and in succession – ventricular tachycardia (VT).
- The atrial electrical activity may fail to pass to the ventricle – heart block.

Cardiac arrhythmias are diagnosed on the basis of history, examination and investigations, including resting electrocardiography (ECG) and 24-hour (or event) monitors.

There are a large number of anti-arrhythmic drugs. Commonly used ones include digoxin for AF, sotalol or amiodarone for paroxysmal AF and β blockers for SVT. Pacemakers are inserted for third degree heart block and symptomatic second degree heart block. Pacemakers are not affected by X-ray machines but strong magnets which are present in MRI scanners may interfere with their function.

Respiratory examination

WIPER (Wash hands, Introduce, Permission, Expose, Reposition)

Position the patient at 45°, and ask them to remove their clothing from above the waist.

Inspection

Look around the bed for clues, eg peak flow meter, inhalers, oxygen masks, sputum pots, non-invasive ventilation machine, chest drain. Scan the patient from head to toe and ask yourself:

- Does the patient look well?
- What is the breathing pattern of the patient, and are they using their accessory muscles of respiration?
- What is their respiratory rate?
- Are they able to talk in complete sentences?
- Are they making any abnormal noises, eg wheeze or stridor?
- What is the colour/ complexion of the patient?

Hands

- Look for: clubbing, peripheral cyanosis, nicotine staining.
- Ask the patient to hold their arms straight out in front of them and spread apart their fingers. The hands may show a tremor which may indicate use of a β_2 adrenoceptor agonist (salbutamol).
- Ask the patient to passively extend the wrists with the arms outstretched – repeated involuntary flexion of the wrists may indicate carbon dioxide retention flap.

Face

- Scan the eyes and look for:
  - ptosis (drooping upper eyelid)
  - miosis (constricted pupil on one side)
  - enophthalmos (a sunken eye).
- The above signs are typical of Horner's syndrome, which may indicate presence of apical lung cancer.
- Inspect the conjunctivae for anaemia.
- Look at the tongue for central cyanosis.

Other
- Examine the radial pulse.
- Examine the cervical lymph nodes.
- Examine the jugulovenous pressure.

Praecordium

Look for:

- chest wall deformities
- scars
- overexpansion.

Palpate

Assess the symmetry of expansion of the chest. Place your hands either side of the midline of the chest with the thumbs touching and ask the patient to breathe in and out. Note how your thumbs move apart with each inspiration.

Percussion

Percuss the praecordium by spreading out the fingers of one hand and resting the palm and fingers on the chest wall. Position your middle finger with the tip in an intercostal space. Strike the middle phalanx of this finger with the middle finger of the other hand. You should practise this again and again.

Percuss the supraclavicular regions, the clavicles, the chest wall in at least six positions and the axillae. Always compare left with right, by assessing both sides at each level. Determine whether the sound is normal, hyper-resonant, dull or stony dull.

Auscultation
- Listen in the same positions which were percussed.
- Ask the patient to inspire deeply and then exhale through the mouth in each position of the stethoscope and describe the sounds and whether there are any extra sounds such as wheeze or crackling.
- Ask the patient to say '99' when you are auscultating. This assesses tactile vocal fremitus.

- Finish the examination by stating that you would like to:
    - look at the temperature chart
    - perform a peak flow reading
    - auscultate the heart.

How to perform a peak expiratory flow measurement (PEFR)

- Ensure that you use a clean mouthpiece for each patient.
- Ask the patient to take a large breath in through the mouth, place their lips around the tube to form a tight seal, and then breathe out as quickly and as forcefully as possible into the meter (as if blowing out birthday cake candles).
- Repeat this three times.
- This shifts the arrow in the gauge and the highest recorded value is noted.
- It is often appropriate to do this before and after treatment with an inhaled bronchodilator.
- The normal PEFR for a patient depends on their height; check the normal value on the chart.
- Dispose of the tube.
- Record your reading on the peak flow chart.

6

Airway Disorders

Normal anatomy and physiology

Respiratory drive is normally maintained by the level of arterial pCO_2. A rise in pCO_2 stimulates an increase in the rate and depth of breathing. Air passes through the large airways (nasopharynx, trachea, bronchi), to the medium-sized airways (bronchioles) and finally into the terminal bronchiole which opens up into the alveolus where gaseous exchange takes place. The majority of resistance to airflow is at the small airways. The airways are lined with ciliated columnar epithelium, goblet cells and muscle cells. The cilia and macrophages are responsible for keeping the airway clear (mucociliary escalator).

The maximum volume of air that can be breathed out is termed the vital capacity. After full expiration some air always remains in the lungs – this is the residual volume.

Total lung capacity = residual volume + vital capacity

The fastest rate of flow achieved during a forced expiration is termed the peak expiratory flow ('peak flow'). The volume of air that can be expired in the first second of a forced expiration is the FEV1.

Hypersecretory chronic bronchitis

Hypersecretory chronic bronchitis is defined as cough, productive of sputum on most days for 3 months over 2 consecutive years. The pathological hallmark is goblet cell hyperplasia. This may occur due to chemical insult to the lungs such as smoking. It is abnormal to have cough productive of significant sputum. As the disease progresses, the patient develops chronic airflow limitation. The FEV1 falls with a rise in residual volume; the FEV1/FVC ratio is reduced and there is shortness of breath on exertion. Most patients adapt to slowly rising arterial pCO_2 and eventually rely on hypoxia to maintain their respiratory drive. It is therefore dangerous to give these patients high concentrations of inspired oxygen since their respiratory drive is abolished and respiratory arrest may occur.

Right-sided heart failure complicates the disorder with the development of ankle swelling and raised jugular venous pressure. The hypoxia results in the clinical signs of central and peripheral cyanosis. These patients are often described as 'blue bloaters'.

Emphysema

Emphysema is defined as destruction of the airways distal to the terminal bronchiole. It often co-exists with hypersecretory chronic bronchitis. Lung function tests show a low FEV1/FVC ratio and a marked reduction in transfer factor. Many patients with emphysema retain sensitivity to rising pCO_2 and become very breathless at last ('pink puffers').

There is considerable clinical overlap between emphysema and chronic bronchitis and patients with these conditions are sometimes described as having chronic obstructive pulmonary disease (COPD).

Patients develop progressive shortness of breath over many years. The gradual decline in respiratory reserve is punctuated with acute exacerbations in which patients may become extremely unwell. Often these are related to super-added chest infections or decompensated heart failure and should be treated with antibiotics and diuretics. Physiotherapy is also important. Many of these patients cannot lie flat and this should be borne in mind when examining or treating them. Patients with a low arterial pO_2 who do not retain pCO_2 (ie pink puffers) can be prescribed home oxygen. There should be no smoking in these households. These patients are poor operative risks. General anaesthesia and ventilation may alter their respiratory drive and post-operative chest infections may be life-threatening.

The British Thoracic Society states that the degree of severity of COPD should be assessed with:

- spirometry
- bronchodilator response
- chest radiograph.

Severity is defined as:

- Mild – if FEV1 is 60–80% predicted
- Moderate – if FEV1 is 40–59% predicted
- Severe – if FEV1 is < 40% predicted.

Treatment

Non-pharmacological
- Stop smoking
- Encourage exercise
- Dietician assessment to aid treatment of obesity
- Influenza/pneumococcal vaccination.

Pharmacological
- Mild – ipratropium inhaled as required.
- Moderate – regular ipratropium or long acting β_2 agonist (salmeterol) with or without inhaled steroid (fluticasone).
- Severe – consider a steroid trial and assess for home nebulisers, and theophyllines.

Asthma

Asthma is a disorder of the small airways, which become hyper-reactive to exogenous stimuli. The muscle around these airways may contract leading to air trapping and low FEV1. Typical triggering factors for an attack are smoke, dust, pets, hairsprays, perfumes and soap powders. Dentists should be aware that a number of chemicals used in the surgery may precipitate asthma in susceptible individuals. In patients with otherwise normal lungs (eg non-smoking teenagers) there may be no sign or symptoms between attacks. During an attack the patient becomes short of breath and wheezy. Lung function tests confirm that the major problem is in expiration (when the wheeze is heard) and there is a reduction in the peak expiratory flow rate (PEFR, peak flows). However, patients often complain of difficulty breathing in because their lungs become hyper-expanded. The attacks are frightening for the patient who may become very anxious. Attacks are often worse in the early morning.

Many patients seem to improve as they get older. However, the disease may appear for the first time in later life (late-onset asthma) or patients may become progressively more short of breath and develop features suggestive of chronic bronchitis or emphysema. In these patients, there is an element of fixed airflow limitation. There is always a varied overlap between reversible and irreversible airflow limitation and therefore some patients with chronic obstructive airways disease (COAD) or emphysema are treated with inhaled bronchodilators or steroids.

Treatment of the acute attack includes oxygen, nebulised bronchodilators (eg Ventolin), steroids and theophyllines. Acute asthma may be a life-threatening condition. Treatment for chronic asthma includes regular use of inhaled steroids, bronchodilators and theophyllines. Severe cases also require systemic steroids, and all such patients should be under the supervision of a chest specialist.

It is important to note that many patients who are prescribed inhalers do not use them correctly and obtain little benefit apart from the placebo effect. Devices are available to improve delivery of the drug (eg volumatics).

The British Thoracic Society's guidelines for the treatment of asthma have five steps:

Step 1 – occasional short-acting β_2 agonist as required for symptom relief. If used more than once daily or there are night time symptoms go to step 2.

Step 2 – add standard dose inhaled steroid, eg beclomethasone. If still symptomatic move to step 3.

Step 3 – Add a long-acting β_2 agonist (salmeterol).

Step 4 – consider oral theophyllines or leukotriene receptor antagonists.

Step 5 – add regular oral prednisolone and refer.

Asthma can be life-threatening, and should always be taken very seriously. In a severe attack:

- the patient is unable to complete sentences
- respiratory rate is > 25 breaths per minute
- pulse rate is > 100 beats per minute
- peak expiratory flow rate is < 50% of best
- there is life-threatening asthma
- peak expiratory flow rate is < 33% of best
- signs include silent chest, cyanosis, poor respiratory effort
- there may be bradycardia
- the patient may appear exhausted or confused or be in coma.

Treatment

- 100% oxygen
- Salbutamol nebulisers
- Hydrocortisone 100 mg iv
- Ipratropium bromide 0.5 mg every 4 hours
- Get help.

Pulmonary fibrosis

A large number of diseases cause fibrosis in the lungs. They tend to present with increasing shortness of breath, first on exertion and then at rest. Unlike COPD, these patients have small scarred lungs with a low Total Lung Capacity (TLC) and Residual Volume (RV). The FEV1 is low but the FEV1/FVC ratio is raised. Cases of pulmonary fibrosis include sarcoidosis, fibrosing alveolitis and it is a side-effect of methotrexate usage. Right heart failure results from pulmonary hypertension.

Extrinsic allergic alveolitis

The extrinsic allergic alveolitis group of disorders eventually results in pulmonary fibrosis due to a hypersensitivity reaction in the lungs. Many occupational lung diseases fall into this category including farmer's lung and bird fancier's lung.

Coal workers' pneumoconiosis

Coalworkers' pneumoconiosis is relatively frequent in South Wales. It is due to the recurrent inhalation of coal dust which leads to pulmonary fibrosis. Pneumoconiosis is classified according to chest radiograph findings into 'simple' and 'complicated'. Compensation is available to sufferers.

Asbestosis

Inhaled asbestos causes pulmonary fibrosis. Specific concerns relate to the risk of carcinoma and mesothelioma, especially in relation to blue asbestos.

Inhaled foreign body

A foreign body may become trapped in the large airways causing sudden respiratory distress and asphyxia. This is a potential problem in dental practice. Heimlich's manoeuvre may dislodge a foreign body. Stand behind the patient, clench one hand and press the fist into the patient's epigastrium with the aid of the other hand and suddenly squeeze the patient, pushing the fist backward and upwards. If this fails, a needle can be inserted between the thyroid and cricoid cartilages.

7
Chest Infections and Lung Cancer

Upper respiratory tract infections

Upper respiratory tract infections (URTIs) are among the most common reasons that people visit their GP. Coryzal symptoms may be because of the common cold, sinusitis and pharyngitis. Many patients describe themselves as having 'flu' but this is a more serious condition associated with systemic upset. Patients with recurrent URTI symptoms may in fact have allergic rhinitis, which will respond better to intranasal steroids than recurrent prescription of antibiotics. Most URTIs are viral and do not require antibiotics. Antibiotics may cause hypersensitivity reactions in these circumstances (eg in glandular fever). Tonsils should be swabbed if an exudate is present.

Streptococcal throat infection may rarely lead to rheumatic fever and penicillin is therefore indicated if the organism is isolated. General anaesthesia for elective surgery should be postponed in the presence of a URTI.

Lower respiratory tract infections

Elderly people and patients with pre-existing lung disease are more prone to lower respiratory tract infection. Patchy infection, usually in the lower lobes, is termed bronchopneumonia. It is a common cause of death in the elderly and a frequent cause of deterioration in patients with COAD. Green sputum may be produced (although this may also be seen in patients with non-infective disease such as asthma).

Lobar pneumonia produces a characteristic clinical picture with an acute pyrexial illness, pleuritic chest pain and dyspnea. Patients may become hypoxic and confused. Green sputum or haemoptysis may also occur. On examination, patients have tachypnoea, crackles in the chest and perhaps pleural rub. Common organisms include *Pneumococcus* and *Haemophilus influenzae* but in around a third of patients the causative organism is never isolated.

'Atypical pneumonia' is the term applied to lower respiratory tract infections caused by such organisms as *Mycoplasma pneumoniae*, *Legionella* and *Coxiella burnetii*. These infections may result in serious systemic upset with renal impairment, hepatic failure and even death.

'Nosocomial' pneumonia is the term applied to hospital-acquired infection (Table 7.1); the causative organisms include Gram-negative and

Gram-positive cocci with varying antibiotic resistance. Immunosuppressed patients (eg due to drugs, acquired immune deficiency syndrome (AIDS)) are at risk of opportunistic infections, eg infections caused by *Pneumocystis carinii*, cytomegalovirus or *Aspergillus*.

At-risk patients, eg diabetic patients and those with pre-existing lung disease, should be encouraged to have the flu vaccination every year. Patients with human immunodeficiency virus (HIV) infection are given prophylactic treatment against *Pneumocystis*. Community-acquired chest infections are typically treated with co-amoxiclav and clarithromycin. Nosocomial infections may be treated with cefuroxime.

The severity of the pneumonia can be assessed using the mnemonic CURB 65:

- Confusion
- Urea > 7 mmol/l
- Respiratory rate > 30 breaths per minute
- Blood pressure < 90 mmHg systolic
- Age > 65 years.

If a patient meets three of the above criteria, the pneumonia is described as severe.

Table 7.1 Various types of pneumonia and their treatment

Bacteria causing pneumonia	Treatment
Community-acquired	
Streptococcus pneumoniae	Amoxicillin 500 mg three times daily and erythromycin 500 mg four times daily
Haemophilus influenzae	
As above but severe	Co-amoxiclav iv or cefuroxime and erythromycin iv
Legionella pneumophila	Clarithromycin 500 mg twice daily
Chlamydia species	Tetracycline
Pneumocystis carinii	High dose co-trimoxazole
Hospital acquired	
Pseudomonas	
Anaerobes	
Gram-negative bacilli	Aminoglycoside iv + cefotaxime
Aspiration	
Streptococcus pneumoniae	
Anaerobes	Cefuroxime and metronidazole

Cystic fibrosis

This is a relatively common autosomal recessive condition in which sufferers inherit a defect in a membrane protein normally expressed on epithelial cells. Several different mutations have been described resulting in a characteristic phenotype of hyperviscous secretions (lung, pancreas).

The condition may present in the neonatal period, manifesting as paralytic ileus, or it may present later in childhood as recurrent chest infections. Despite prophylactic antibiotics and regular postural drainage (with physiotherapy), the lungs become chronically infected and scarred.

Pulmonary tuberculosis

Tuberculosis may affect many parts of the body and is caused by a variety of mycobacteria. With increasing affluence, the incidence of pulmonary tuberculosis in the UK had been declining, but it is now becoming more common again, especially among homeless and immunosuppressed people and immigrants. Primary infection may occur in childhood with few or no clinical features, leaving a scarred area in the periphery of the lung or at the apex and perhaps some calcified lymph nodes. The disease reactivates in later life when conditions allow. 'Open' cases release infective mycobacteria in sputum and are a public health hazard. The disease may present insidiously with lethargy, malaise, weight loss, fever and sweats. Changing shadows occur on the chest radiograph and the mycobacterium may be isolated in sputum.

Pulmonary tuberculosis is treated with multiple agents (eg rifampicin, isoniazid and ethambutol) for 6–9 months. Treatment no longer requires long periods of hospitalisation and the main concern is one of ensuring patient compliance with the medication as an out-patient. Tuberculosis may also present as: miliary tuberculosis, tubercular meningitis, genitourinary tuberculosis, osteomyelitis, peritonitis and pericarditis.

Lung cancer

Bronchial carcinoma is the most common malignancy in the UK, accounting for over 30 000 deaths a year. Risk factors include smoking and asbestos exposure. The majority are squamous cell cancers that arise in squamous dysplastic areas of normal columnar epithelium. Common presenting symptoms include cough, haemoptysis, dyspnoea and chest wall discomfort. If the cancer occludes a medium-sized airway, collapse and superadded infection occurs in the part of the lung distal to the obstruction. Occlusion of a main bronchus results in severe shortness of breath. Lung cancer may also present with systemic upset, weight loss and malaise or signs of superior vena cava obstruction. Metastases occur in bone, brain or liver. Some tumours secrete hormones, leading to the development of Cushing's syndrome or syndrome of inappropriate antidiuretic hormone secretion with hyponatraemia. Apart from signs in the chest, physical examination may reveal finger clubbing and Horner's syndrome (ptosis, constricted pupil).

Besides squamous cell bronchial carcinoma, other histological types include oat cell (25%) and large cell (20%) cancers and adenocarcinoma (20%). Many lung cancers are inoperable at the time of presentation. Palliative treatment with radiotherapy is the most common treatment, although chemotherapy may be useful, especially in oat cell cancers.

Mesothelioma

This is a tumour of the pleural lining in the lung. It is relatively uncommon but its importance lies in the strong association with previous asbestos exposure. Patients present with malignant pleural effusion and the diagnosis is made by pleural biopsy. Compensation is available to victims.

8
Tubular Gut

Oesophagus

Disorders of the oesophagus often present with difficulty swallowing (dysphagia). Unless it is associated with a sore throat or oropharyngeal ulceration, dysphagia is a serious symptom that requires investigation. Causes of dysphagia include:

- cancer: pharynx, oesophagus, stomach, lung
- benign strictures: reflux, foreign body, swallowing corrosives
- neurological: bulbar palsy, myasthenia gravis
- motility disorders: achalasia, corkscrew oesophagus.

Gastro-oesophageal reflux disease is a common disorder due to the gastro-oesophageal junction being above the diaphragm. Patients may have severe symptoms of heartburn and acid reflux. Alcohol, caffeine and tobacco all relax the sphincter and may contribute to symptoms. Treatment includes losing weight, antacids and proton pump blockers such as omeprazole.

Stomach

Disorders may present with dysphagia, vomiting, haematemesis or weight loss. Cancer of the stomach may cause all of these symptoms and unless diagnosed early, the prognosis is poor.

Peptic ulcer disease affects mainly the stomach and duodenum. Normally, a protective mucosal barrier prevents the peptic acids from damaging the lining of the upper gastrointestinal tract. When this fails, peptic ulceration results and may present with burning (dyspeptic) pain. Chronic iron deficiency anaemia may result from slow, clinically inapparent bleeding from the ulcers. Brisker bleeding may result in haematemesis or melaena, both of which require urgent admission to hospital. Other causes of haematemesis include oesophageal varices and Mallory–Weiss tears.

Duodenal ulceration has been associated with *Helicobacter pylori* infection in the gastric antrum. The organism may be responsible for increased acid secretion and attempts are often made to eradicate *H. pylori* in patients with chronic ulceration. This may prove difficult and reinfection often occurs. The organism has been found in the mouths of such patients and this may represent a source of recolonisation of the stomach and duodenum.

The upper gastrointestinal tract may be investigated by endoscopy, barium swallow or meal and occasionally pH studies.

Peptic disease is treated with antacids, H2 blockers (cimetidine, ranitidine) or proton pump blockers such as omeprazole.

The small bowel

Many disorders of the small bowel will present with malabsorption. The two most common are coeliac disease (gluten enteropathy) and Crohn's disease. Other causes of malabsorption include bacterial overgrowth, previous surgical resection and exocrine pancreatic failure (eg cystic fibrosis).

Coeliac disease

Coeliac disease results from hypersensitivity to the gliadin fraction of gluten-containing foods (wheat, rye, barley and oats). Exposed patients develop flat (atrophic) duodenal villi and malabsorption with diarrhoea, bloating and weight loss. Although many cases are diagnosed in infancy, symptoms may arise at any age or the disease may be suspected following the incidental discovery of iron or folate deficiency. The diagnosis is confirmed by duodenal biopsy at endoscopy. Treatment is with a gluten-free diet. Patients with coeliac disease who continue to consume gluten are at increased risk of small bowel lymphoma.

Crohn's disease

Crohn's disease is a chronic disease of uncertain aetiology. It may affect any part of the intestine from mouth (aphthous ulcers) to anus, but the most common sites are the terminal ileum and colon. Focal inflammation with fissures, ulcers and giant cell granulomas develop with healthy intestine between the lesions (skip lesions). Patients may present with fever, diarrhoea, abdominal pain, weight loss and failure to thrive. Anal and perianal fistulae and skin tags are characteristic features; other extraintestinal features include arthritis, uveitis and skin rashes. The disease progresses with relapses and remissions and may be treated with oral steroids. Severe relapses require admission to hospital for intravenous steroids, fluids and antibiotics.

The large bowel (colon)

Ulcerative colitis

Together with Crohn's disease, ulcerative colitis makes up the clinical entity of inflammatory bowel disease. In some patients it is difficult to distinguish between two diagnoses. However, ulcerative colitis usually affects the large bowel starting at the rectum and proceeding proximally (i.e. no skip lesions). Only 10% of patients with ulcerative colitis have terminal ileal disease (backwash ileitis). Histologically, Crohn's and ulcerative colitis can usually be distinguished by an experienced histopathologist. Ulcerative colitis presents with bloody diarrhoea (> 7 days duration), sweats, fever, weight loss, and sometimes florid aphthous ulcers. Treatment is with rectal steroids, sulphasalazine and oral steroids.

Severe relapses of inflammatory bowl disease may produce an 'acute abdomen' termed toxic megacolon. If this does not settle with intravenous steroids and fluids, surgical resection may be required. There is an increased risk of colonic malignancy, especially in patients with longstanding ulcerative colitis.

Carcinoma of the colon

Colonic cancer is a common malignancy responsible for more than 15 000 deaths per year in the UK. Predisposing causes include a positive family history, familial polyposis and inflammatory bowel disease. Colonic cancers are more common on the left side of the colon and can grow silently, presenting late with intestinal obstruction or metastases. They may cause iron deficiency anaemia by slow bleeding. More rapid bleeding results in frank rectal bleeding (melaena is more suggestive of an upper gastrointestinal cause). Rectal tumours can be felt by palpation. The stage of the disease may be classified by Dukes' criteria and this gives an indication of prognosis. Treatment is surgical.

Patients with ulcerative colitis or familial polyposis should undergo regular colonoscopy screening for malignancy.

Irritable bowel syndrome

This is a very common condition. Patients complain of colicky abdominal pains, sometimes relieved by bowel action. Intermittent diarrhoea or constipation may also be features. These symptoms may also indicate carcinoma of the colon so many patients undergo investigations including barium enema of colonoscopy. Although these tests are normal in irritable bowel syndrome, many patients remain anxious about their symptoms; flare-ups may coincide with periods of stress. Treatment includes a high-fibre diet, antispasmodics and reassurance.

Diverticular disease

Diverticula are outpouchings of the colon – typically in left side of colon. Diverticula are a common finding on barium enemas and are normally asymptomatic. However, they may cause acute abdominal pain if they become infected (diverticulitis) and may also be a source of rectal bleeding.

Examination of the abdomen

1. WIPER (Wash hands, Introduce, Permission, Expose, Reposition)
2. Inspect from the front of the bed.
3. Inspect the hands: look for finger clubbing, anaemia, leukonychia (white nails), palmar erythema, Dupuytren's contracture.
4. Inspect the face: look for xanthelasma and corneal arcus.
5. Inspect the conjunctiva for anaemia and look at the sclera for jaundice.
6. Look in the mouth for ulcers.
7. Look at the thorax and arms for spider naevi.
8. Inspect the abdomen: look for swelling, distended veins, skin changes, scars, herniae, pulsation, stomas.
9. Superficial palpation of the abdomen.
10. Deep palpation of the abdomen: palpate for the liver, spleen, kidneys, aorta.
11. Percuss the abdomen for shifting dullness (ascites).
12. Auscultate the abdomen.
13. Thank the patient.

Examiners' favourites

What are the causes of a distended abdomen?
Answer: 'The 6 Fs': fat, fluid (ascites), fetus, flatus, faeces and flipping great tumour.

9

Liver and Pancreatic Disease

Functions of the normal liver

- Synthesis of proteins
    - albumin
    - coagulation factors
    - iron binding proteins
    - protease inhibitors.
- Detoxification of drugs and toxins
- Bile production:
    - bile acids
    - cholesterol
    - bilirubin (product of haemoglobin metabolism).

Symptoms and signs of liver disease

Jaundice (icterus)

Jaundice occurs due to excess bilirubin in the blood and is detectable clinically at levels greater than approximately three times the normal. It is caused by either obstruction to bile flow from the liver or by damage to liver cells (hepatocellular jaundice) resulting in an inability to secrete bilirubin.

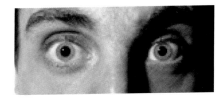

Figure 9.1 The sclera in jaundice.

Coagulopathy

Poor blood clotting may occur due to an inability to absorb vitamin K which, being fat soluble, requires normal bile flow for absorption. Vitamin K is required to synthesise clotting factors II, VII, IX and X. Coagulopathy may also occur due to increased protein production in cases of severe hepatocellular damage.

Encephalopathy

There is decreased level of consciousness – initially may be mild lack of concentration but may progress to coma.

Ascites

Fluid retention in the abdomen in multifactorial:

- decreased plasma oncotic pressure due to low albumin
- increased fluid retention due to decreased liver metabolism of the mineralocorticoid aldosterone
- increased portal venous pressure due to obstruction of the portal blood flow in the liver because of fibrosis.

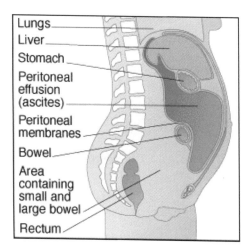

Lungs
Liver
Stomach
Peritoneal effusion (ascites)
Peritoneal membranes
Bowel
Area containing small and large bowel
Rectum

Figure 9.2. Ascites leads to distension of the abdomen and can compress the organs.

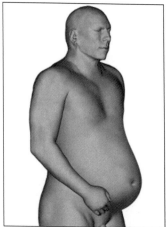

Figure 9.3. Typical appearance of ascites.

Portal hypertension

Increased portal blood pressure leads to engorgement of the spleen with blood and a syndrome of hypersplenism where blood cells, particularly platelets, are used up in the spleen. The low platelet count aggravates any bleeding tendency. Blood drains via alternative pathways avoiding the liver giving rise to enlarged veins at the lower end of the oesophagus, which can rupture and bleed catastrophically.

Laboratory liver function tests

- Aspartate aminotransferase (AST) levels are increased in hepatocellular damage, eg alcohol, paracetamol overdose.
- Alkaline phosphatase increased in obstructive jaundice, eg gallstones.
- Bilirubin increased in both hepatocellular damage and obstructive jaundice.
- Albumin decreased in chronic liver disease.
- Gamma glutamyl transferase increased in obstructive jaundice but commonly used to assess alcohol intake as it is induced by alcohol consumption.
- International normalised ratio is prolonged in severe hepatocellular damage.

Causes of acute liver disease

- Acute viral hepatitis
- Paracetamol overdose – commonest cause in UK of severe acute liver failure
- Acute fatty liver
- Alcoholic hepatitis
- Drugs, eg halothane.

Some causes of chronic liver disease

- Hepatitis B
- Hepatitis C
- Alcohol
- Primary biliary cirrhosis
- Autoimmune chronic active hepatitis
- Alpha$_1$ antitrypsin deficiency
- Haemochromatosis
- Wilson's disease.

Viral hepatitis

Hepatitis A

- Commonest in children
- Spread by faecal–oral route
- Incidence declining due to better hygiene
- Increase incidence in institutions and among drug misusers
- Incubation period 4–6 weeks
- Rarely causes liver failure
- Never causes chronic liver disease
- Characterised by a gastrointestinal upset with or without jaundice
- Diagnosed by detecting IgM antibodies in the serum.

Hepatitis B (HB)

- Parenteral transmission, virus detected in blood, semen, saliva and urine.
- Commonest route of transmission worldwide is transplacental.
- Virus can survive in dried blood.
- Virus is inactivated by 2 minutes 98°C or by 60 minutes in 2% glutaraldehyde solution.
- Incidence has not altered in UK despite current immunisation regimen.
- Incubation period is 2–6 months.
- Less than 10% of infected people develop acute liver failure in the UK.
- 10–15% become chronic carriers (higher if transmitted transplacentally).
- 10–15% chronic carriers develop hepatocellular carcinoma.

Pattern of antigen/antibody test in Hepatitis B

Patient has had recent infection:

- No HB surface (HBs) antibody yet
- HB core IgM still positive.

Patient has had infection and is no longer infectious:

- HBs antibody positive
- HBs antigen negative
- HBe antibody positive.

Patient has been immunised:

- HBs antibody positive
- HBs antigen negative
- HBe antibody negative.

Patient is a chronic carrier:

- HBs antigen positive
- HBs antibody negative
- HBe antibody positive.

Patient is a highly infectious carrier:

- HBs antigen positive
- HBs antibody negative
- HBe antigen positive
- HBe antibody negative.

Treatment

Interferon alfa is useful in those who have active disease particularly those who are e antigen positive. HB infection is no longer an absolute contraindication to liver transplantation.

Prevention
- Worldwide carrier rates may be higher than 7%.
- The only effective way of preventing the disease is mass immunisation especially in highly endemic areas such as the Far East and Africa.
- Worldwide hepatocellular carcinoma associated with hepatitis B is the commonest preventable cancer.

Hepatitis C
- Parenteral transmission, especially via blood products.
- There is little evidence for sexual transmission.
- There is high rate of progression to cirrhosis (30–65%).
- Accurate diagnostic tests based on polymerase chain reaction (PCR) technology are now available.
- Most patients are asymptomatic for many years.
- The UK government is now embarking on 'look back' exercise to detect those that may have post-transfusion hepatitis C infection so the apparent frequency will rise.
- Treatment with interferon is only successful in 25% of cases.

Liver transplantation

Indications

- Acute liver failure, eg paracetamol overdose
- Acute fatty liver of pregnancy
- Chronic liver disease, eg primary biliary cirrhosis, alcoholic liver disease
- Neonatal biliary atresia.

Post-operative problems

- Rejection
- Immunosuppression
- Graft-versus-host disease (early signs include oral ulceration).

Obstructive jaundice

Bile flows from the right and left lobes of the liver to the gut via the gallbladder.

Obstruction to bile flow = jaundice.

Causes

- Gallstones, which are commonly associated with abdominal pain.
- Bile duct strictures, which may be benign or malignant
- Pancreatic tumours (always malignant).

10
Diabetes Mellitus

Diabetes mellitus represents a group of disorders characterised by raised blood glucose concentration and deranged metabolism. Diabetes is common and sufferers are at increased risk of cardiovascular, renal, neurological and ophthalmic complications. The disorders can be broadly classified into:

- type 1 diabetes (autoimmune, insulin dependent)
- type 2 (non autoimmune, non-insulin dependent).

Type 1 diabetes

Type 1 diabetes is associated with human leukocyte antigen DR3 and DR4. In this condition there is an autoimmune attack against the β cells in the pancreatic islets, which are destroyed. Although the destruction may occur over months or even years, patients tend to present acutely with a history of only a few days or weeks. Type 1 diabetes may affect any age group (neonates to the elderly), but most patients present in late teenage or early adult life.

Pathophysiology

Destruction of the β cells results in an absolute lack of insulin. Blood glucose rises since insulin is required to metabolise glucose in peripheral cells such as muscle and fat cells. Furthermore, endogenous glucose production is not switched off. As the blood rises, the concentration exceeds the renal threshold for glucose and glucose appears in the urine (glycosuria). The glycosuria produces an osmotic diuresis resulting in polyuria, polydipsia and nocturia. Accumulation of acidic ketone bodies (eg acetoacetic acid) can cause metabolic acidosis. Patients become dehydrated and comatose; the increased ketone levels can cause the breath to have a typically sweet smell and there may be signs of superimposed infection. If the condition is not treated, the person will die.

Emergency treatment

Emergency treatment is with fluid replacement and insulin. The patient would have lost isotonic fluid, which is therefore replaced with normal saline. The patient may have > 10 litre deficit and this needs to be replaced vigorously; however, concerns have been raised regarding excessive fluid replacement and management is tailored to individual patients based on the results of central pressure monitoring, pH, electrolytes and clinical response. Insulin is given intravenously and the dose is titrated according to frequent blood sugar estimations. Once the glucose has fallen to < 14 mmol/l, the fluid is changed from normal saline solution to dextrose; this allows continued infusion of insulin without rendering the patient hypoglycaemic. Intravenous insulin is continued for 24–48 hours to allow metabolism of excessive ketones to continue.

Long-term treatment

Patients with type 1 diabetes will require long-term treatment with insulin. Without insulin, patients will relapse into diabetic ketoacidosis. It is relatively easy to prevent this severe complication occurring – far more difficult is to achieve blood glucose concentrations in the normal range. There is clear evidence that the higher the prevailing blood glucose, the more likely long-term diabetic complications are to develop. The key to good diabetic control is a regular and healthy diet. Dietary advice for people with diabetes has been much simplified in recent years. In essence the diabetic diet is the same as a healthy diet for the general population. Rapidly absorbed carbohydrates such as refined sugars should be avoided since they result in sharp swings in blood glucose. None of the available insulin regimens can mimic the rapid rise and fall of blood glucose following ingestion of a pure carbohydrate load. Patients with diabetes are at greatly increased risk of atheroma, and therefore their diet should be low in fat.

Long-term insulin is given by subcutaneous injection. All insulins come in a standard strength (U100), and may be administered using an insulin syringe or a variety of pen devices. The pen devices remove the need for drawing up the insulin on each occasion. Most patients are on regimens of between two and four injections of insulin a day. Fast-acting, soluble, clear insulin (eg Actrapid, Humulin S) is taken 30 minutes before a meal and has a duration of action of around 4 hours. Manufacturers add a variety of agents including protamine and zinc to clear insulin to produce insulins that have slower onset of action but a longer duration (eg Monotard, Humulin I). These longer-acting insulins are cloudy. Many patients achieve control by self-injecting different proportions of fast- and medium-acting insulin twice a day.

Patients with diabetes need to be aware of their blood glucose levels if they are to make appropriate changes to their insulin dosage. Glycosuria is only a crude estimate of blood glucose concentrations so most patients check their blood glucose levels directly using some sort of stick, eg BM stick. The colour change on the stick indicated the blood glucose concentration and this can read either by eye or using a monitor.

Factors predisposing to type 1 diabetes

- Drugs – steroids and thiazides.
- Pancreatic disease – chronic pancreatitis, cystic fibrosis, surgery.
- Endocrine disease – Cushing's, acromegaly, thyrotoxicosis.
- Others – acanthosis nigrans.

Rules for managing type 1 diabetes

- Patients must never stop their insulin. If they are ill and not eating, they need to check their blood glucose levels frequently, as they may need more, not less, insulin.
- Arrange surgery in diabetic patients for first thing in the morning. Ask patients to take their normal insulin the night before, but to reduce any long-acting insulin by 50–75%. If a patient is to have a general anaesthetic, set up an intravenous line once the patient is nil by mouth and infuse 5% dextrose at a minimum rate of 500 ml 4 hourly. In a separate syringe driver, add 50 units of clear insulin to 50 ml of saline and run between 1 units and 4 units/hour depending on the blood glucose values which should be measured at least hourly. If the patient becomes hypoglycaemic, change the dextrose to 10% or 20%. Only switch off the insulin if patients have BM < 3 mmol/l, and then aim to restart the insulin at 0.5 U/h as soon as the blood glucose rises. There are a number of other regimens for covering patients having surgery; if in doubt, contact the diabetes team in the hospital.
- Patients having procedures under local anaesthesia should take their normal insulin and normal meals. If by lunch-time the patient cannot tolerate food, they are at risk of becoming hypoglycaemic if they have taken long-acting insulin before breakfast – this can usually be overcome by a small glass of sugared milk.
- Inappropriate behaviour, sweating, collapse or coma of rapid onset in any diabetic patient should be treated as hypoglycaemia. Place patient in recovery position and clear airway. Administer glucose – if the patient cannot swallow, use Hypostop gel. If the patient is unconscious, administer 20–50% dextrose iv fast 50–100 ml (and/or glucagon im – if iv access fails). The dextrose iv harms veins so this should be followed by 0.9% saline flush. Expect prompt recovery. If this does not happen, give dexamethasone to combat cerebral oedema after prolonged hypoglycaemia.

Type 2 diabetes

Type 2 diabetes is far more common than type 1 diabetes. Most patients are middle-aged and overweight although the disorder can occur in the young and thin. The problem in type 2 diabetes is a relative lack of insulin but not an absolute deficiency. The relative lack is exacerbated by insulin resistance. The disease often presents insidiously. The blood glucose rises slowly over many months or years and often the patients are diagnosed by chance when a blood glucose level is taken as part of a health scan. When the blood glucose rises sufficiently, patients will develop similar symptoms to those with type 1 diabetes although ketoacidosis is unusual. Since the disease progresses silently, patients may present with established diabetic complications after years of unrecognised moderate hyperglycaemia.

Treatment is aimed at improving insulin sensitivity by diet and exercise. Unfortunately, many patients find it impossible to lose weight. Insulin secretion may be enhanced by a variety of drugs including those sulphonylureas (glibenclamide) and the biguanides (metformin). In some patients the blood glucose continues to rise despite maximum doses of oral hypoglycaemic agents and they are eventually treated with insulin. These patients are best described as having type 2 diabetes requiring insulin.

- Sulphonylureas: stimulate insulin action and insulin sensitivity.
    - tolbutamide – short acting, useful in elderly
    - glibenclamide – intermediate action
    - chlorpropamide – long acting, once a day; avoid in renal impairment.
- Biguanides: improve insulin sensitivity but do not stimulate secretion. Also inhibit hepatic glucoses genesis and often induce anorexia and diarrhoea. Good for obese people as an adjunct. Avoid in hepatic and renal impairment.
- Glitazones: rosiglitazone causes reduced insulin resistance.
- Alpha glucosidase inhibitor: acarbose causes decreased conversion of starch to sugar.

Since diabetic ketoacidosis is not a feature of type 2 diabetes, management of these patients during surgical procedures is relatively straightforward. Most patients can simply omit their oral hypoglycaemic agents on the day of their operation and then restart them once they are eating again. Some patients with high blood glucose levels may be treated with iv insulin and dextrose, especially if they are particularly unwell or are likely to have prolonged surgery and recovery. It is important to note that patients taking tablets for diabetes may also develop hypoglycaemia.

Diabetic complications

These complications are seen in patients with both type 1 and type 2 diabetes.

Eyes

Patients with diabetes develop cataracts at a younger age than the general population. Large swings of blood sugar (osmotic changes) will alter the shape of the lens and cause reversible visual impairment due to refractory errors. Diabetic retinopathy (haemorrhages, exudates, infarcts) may lead to blindness. Early changes may be effectively treated by laser photocoagulation and therefore all patients with diabetes should have their eyes examined at least once a year.

Kidneys

Patients with diabetes may develop diabetic nephropathy. There is thickening of the glomerular mesangium, proteinuria and eventual renal failure. Progression to renal failure may be slowed by tight control of blood pressure.

- Angiotensin-converting enzyme (ACE) inhibitors – enalapril aids insulin sensitivity and may protect against renal disease.
- 25% of young people with diabetes develop chronic renal failure before age 30.

Cardiovascular system

Atheroma is more common and widespread in patients with diabetes. The incidence of heart attacks (three to five times more common), strokes (twice as common), peripheral vascular disease is increased. Advise patients to reduce the risk factors. Treat hypertension vigorously with enalapril.

Nervous system

A variety of neuropathies occur in patients with diabetes including chronic sensory peripheral neuropathy, compression neuropathy, proximal motor neuropathies and autonomic neuropathies. The cause is not known but ischaemia and altered cellular sodium permeability have been suggested.

Autonomic neuropathy

- Postural hypotension
- Nocturnal diarrhoea
- Urinary retention
- Impotence.

Somatic neuropathy

- Symmetric sensory polyneuropathy – distal numbness, tingling and pain, usually worse at night.
- Mononeuritis multiplex – especially affects cranial nerves III and VI.
- Amyotrophy:
    - painful wasting of quadriceps
    - reversible.
    - diabetic foot
    - feet affected by combination of peripheral neuropathy and peripheral vascular disease = numbness, tingling, burning sensation, deformity and high risk of ulceration
    - surgery if: abscesses, osteomyelitis, gangrene, suppurative arthritis, spreading infection.

Hypoglycaemia

This is a common complication of therapy.

11
Pituitary Gland and Gonads

Normal anatomy and physiology

The normal pituitary gland lies in the pituitary fossa in close proximity to the optic chiasm. It is composed of the anterior lobe, intermediate lobe (rudimentary in humans) and the posterior lobe. The anterior lobe is responsible for the secretion of prolactin, growth hormone, adrenocorticotropic hormone (ACTH), thyroid-stimulating hormone (TSH), luteinising hormone (LH) and follicle-stimulating hormone (FSH). The posterior pituitary secretes antidiuretic hormone (ADH) and oxytocin. Pituitary hormones are released as a response to messages from the hypothalamus (eg corticotrophin-releasing hormone (CRH) stimulates ACTH release). The exception is prolactin, the secretion of which is under tonic inhibition mediated by dopamine.

Pituitary gland enlargement

The most common reason the pituitary enlarges is pregnancy. Pathological enlargement can occur as a result of tumour growth in the gland. These tumours are almost always benign in the sense that they do not metastasise. However, because of the position of the pituitary, enlargement can lead to serious consequences. The most common tumour of the pituitary is a non-functioning adenoma but other tumours will secrete functioning hormones (see below).

Pituitary enlargement will encroach on the optic chiasm causing a typical field loss – bitemporal hemianopia. Enlargement may cause other visual disturbances including flashing lights or total uni-ocular blindness. An enlarging pituitary may also produce headaches. If an infarct develops in the gland, the patient presents acutely with headache, sudden visual loss, unwell, hypotensive (pituitary apoplexy).

Hyperprolactinaemia

A raised prolactin level is a common finding, especially in women (in men it presents late as impotence) who may initially present with amenorrhoea or galactorrhoea. In some cases a well-defined pituitary adenoma is found on magnetic resonance imaging (MRI). Sometimes the adenoma is very small (microadenoma) or not visible at all on scanning. Raised prolactin levels can also occur with large pituitary tumours that cause compression of the pituitary stalk and release prolactin secretion from the tonic inhibition of dopamine and certain antidopaminergic drugs. Isolated raised prolactin may require no treatment. However, if galactorrhoea is a problem or periods are irregular with low oestrogen, prolactin levels may be reduced by treating with dopamine agonists such as bromocriptine or cabergoline. The contraceptive pill is sometimes prescribed.

Growth hormone excess

Growth hormone excess is due to a growth-hormone-producing tumour of the pituitary. In childhood this will lead to gigantism. Once the epiphyses are fused in adults it leads to acromegaly with enlargement of the peripheries. Shoe size increases, rings become tight, the tongue enlarges with spaces between the teeth. The skin is oily and coarse. Diabetes or impaired glucose tolerance results. Treatment is by surgery and sometimes somatostatin injections.

ACTH excess

ACTH drives the adrenal to produce too much glucocorticoid. This results in pituitary-dependent Cushing's (Cushing's disease). The pituitary lesion may be small. The differential diagnosis lies between a primary adrenal cause or ectopic ACTH syndrome. Patients develop typical cushingoid features with moon face, buffalo hump, easy bruising, hypertension, diabetes, osteoporosis, myopathy, hypokalaemia, wasting of tissues, thin skin and purple striae.

TSH, LH, FSH

Pituitary lesions causing excessive levels of these hormones are rare.

ADH excess

Excessive production of ADH results in the syndrome of inappropriate ADH secretion. Urine is concentrated and plasma is diluted with low serum sodium. The condition may be the result of head injury, pituitary surgery or secondary systemic disease such as pneumonia.

Pituitary hormone deficiency

Isolated pituitary hormone deficiency may arise. Clinically important
are deficiency of growth hormone (dwarfism), and LH and FSH
(hypogonadotropic hypogonadism). More often a range of defects are found,
eg after the pituitary has been removed surgically or if normal function is
impaired by a tumour. Hormones require to be replaced as follows:

1. ACTH – replace with steroids (hydrocortisone)
2. TSH – replace with thyroxine
3. LH/FSH – replace with oestrogen or testosterone
4. Growth hormone – sometimes replaced
5. Prolactin – never replaced
6. ADH – replace with nasal spray.

Ovaries

These respond to cyclical changes in LH and FSH to produce oestrogens
(mainly oestradiol), progesterone and monthly ovulation. A variety of tumours
may arise in the ovaries, some of which are malignant. Disordered ovulatory
function in women is common and has a large number of causes, including
stress, weight loss or gain and pituitary disease. Hirsutism is a common
complaint and, although it may be due to androgen-secreting tumours,
is usually benign and self-limiting. Premature ovarian failure may result
from a primary (autoimmune) disease or as a result of surgical removal of
both ovaries. Hormone replacement therapy is given to prevent premature
osteoporosis as a result of oestrogen deficiency.

Testes

Testes respond to LH and FSH to produce androgens (mainly testosterone)
and spermatogenesis. Testicular cancer is relatively common in young men
and presents with painless swelling. Testicular failure is treated with monthly
testosterone injections. Oral preparations are less reliable. Androgens and
anabolic steroids are liable to misuse. This results in testicular atrophy.

12
Thyroid and Adrenals

Thyroid gland

Normal physiology

The thyroid gland consists of two lobes and an isthmus, and lies in the neck. Rarely the only functioning thyroid tissue is in the oral cavity (lingual thyroid). A normal thyroid gland can just be palpated as soft tissue in front of the trachea. The thyroid gland concentrates iodine from the diet and incorporates it into thyroglobulin. The gland then secretes thyroxine (T_4). The activity of the thyroid is regulated by thyroid-stimulating hormone (TSH) which is produced by the pituitary gland. T_4 is then converted into its active metabolite T_3. Raised levels of T_3 inhibit TSH release while if the T_3 level falls, TSH production is enhanced. Thus a feedback loop exists to maintain levels of T_3.

Hypothyroidism

Congenital hypothyroidism

Children are sometimes born with hypothyroidism, either because the thyroid gland is missing or an inherited enzyme defect blocks the production of T_4. Untreated, this leads to stunting of growth but most importantly, mental impairment (cretinism). All children have thyroid-stimulating hormone (TSH) levels measured in the second week of life as a screening process. If TSH is high, T_4 is estimated and treatment commenced as required.

Acquired hypothyroidism

There are many causes of hypothyroidism including:

- having surgery
- having radioiodine therapy
- over-use of antithyroid drugs
- primary autoimmune disorder
- Hashimoto's disease
- drug induced – amiodarone
- secondary to pituitary failure.

Clinical features

- Tiredness
- Lethargy
- Weight gain
- Constipation
- Irregular and heavy periods
- Cold intolerance
- Dry skin and hair
- Puffiness of skin.

Patients may have a scar of previous thyroid surgery, a goitre or slow relaxing ankle jerks.

Treatment

This involves thyroxine (T_4). Usually the drug is given once a day and the dose is adjusted to maintain normal T_4 and TSH levels.

Hyperthyroidism (thyrotoxicosis)

Excessive T_4 may be due to a number of reasons, including:

- over-treatment with T_4
- Graves' disease
- single toxic nodule
- toxic multinodular goitre
- amiodarone
- self-administration of thyroxine.

Clinical features

Weight loss despite good appetite, diarrhoea, heat intolerance, jittery, tremor, myopathy, resting tachycardia, palmar erythema, lid retraction. Patients with Graves' disease frequently have other signs – exophthalmos, diplopia and pretibial myxoedema.

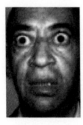

Figure 12.1 Exophthalmos.

Treatment

- Drugs – carbimazole, propranolol
- Radioiodine
- Surgery.

Thyroid cancer

Lumps in the neck may be thyroid cancer. This is potentially curable and can occur in relatively young patients and therefore all patients with thyroid nodules should be investigated. This is usually done by ultrasound followed by fine needle aspiration of thyroid nodule. Thyroid cancers include papillary, follicular and anaplastic cancers. Treatment is usually surgical, together with radioiodine.

Adrenal glands

The adrenal glands lie above the kidneys. They produce glucocorticoid, mineralocorticoid and androgen hormones. Glucocorticoid (cortisol) secretion is under the control of ACTH, which is secreted by the anterior pituitary gland. Mineralocorticoid (aldosterone) secretion is under the control of the renin–angiotensin system. Adrenal function is essential for life.

Excessive glucocorticoid secretion

Excessive glucocorticoid secretion results in the clinical picture of Cushing's syndrome. Causes include a pituitary adenoma secreting ACTH (Cushing's disease), an adrenal adenoma secreting cortisol, an ectopic source of ACTH (eg lung cancer), bilateral adrenal hyperplasia or exogenous administration or pharmacological doses of steroids (eg in asthma). Clinical features include:

- Weight gain (centripetal)
- Moon face
- Buffalo hump
- Easy bruising
- Thin skin
- Proximal myopathy
- Hypertension
- Diabetes
- Osteopetrosis
- Acne
- Striae.

It can be very difficult to decide the cause of Cushing's syndrome. Investigations include urinary free cortisol, plasma cortisol following dexamethasone administration, ACTH levels, chest radiograph, magnetic resonance imaging (MRI) of adrenals and pituitary glands, and selective venous sampling for ACTH.

Inadequate glucocorticoid secretion

Inadequate glucocorticoid secretion may be due to pituitary gland failure (lack of ACTH – only glucocorticoids lacking) or failure/destruction of both adrenal glands (all adrenal hormones lacking). The latter may be due to autoimmune destruction and is termed Addison's disease. This is a life-threatening condition. Patients may present insidiously with malaise, tiredness, lethargy, weight loss and hypotension. If the adrenals have failed, there is pigmentation due to excessive pituitary ACTH secretion (in an attempt to compensate for the lack of cortisol). Patients are at risk of circulatory collapse during an intercurrent illness or stress, eg being under anaesthesia. Urgent treatment with replacement steroids (hydrocortisone with or without fludrocortisone) is required. This treatment is lifelong. Patients are given a card to carry giving information about diagnosis and treatment. Replacement steroid dose should be tripled during acute illness. Steroids must be given iv in hospital if they cannot be taken orally. Extra doses are given with pre-medication and during surgery.

Patients on long-term pharmacological doses of steroids develop adrenal insufficiency because the pituitary–adrenal axis 'goes to sleep'. Long-term steroid therapy must never be stopped suddenly. A collapsed patient known to be on steroids must be given iv hydrocortisone as part of resuscitation measures.

Excessive mineralocorticoid secretion

Excessive mineralocorticoid secretion may be due to an aldosterone-secreting adrenal adenoma. It causes hypertension associated with hypokalaemia (Conn's syndrome).

Excessive adrenal androgen secretion

Some adrenal tumours secrete androgens resulting in virilisation in females. The major source of androgens in males are the testes.

Examination of a thyroid gland

1. WIPER (Wash hands, Introduce, Permission, Expose, Reposition)
2. Inspect from the end of the bed. Look for clues of other disease. Does the patient have obvious signs of Graves' disease? What is their weight like?
3. Are their hands warm, cold, sweaty? Is there a tremor?
4. Inspect the radial pulse.
5. Measure the blood pressure.
6. Inspect the eyes and face. Look for exophthalmos. Look for peaches and cream complexion.
7. Assess eye movements. Inspect the eyes from above and from the sides. Watch for lid lag and retraction.
8. Inspect the neck. Look at the patient from the side and from the front, with the tongue in the mouth, protruded, and during swallowing. A thyroglossal cyst will move superiorly on swallowing.
9. Palpate the neck. Stand behind the patient and palpate the whole thyroid gland. Stabilise the lateral lobe with one hand, and palpate the other lobe with the other hand. Repeat with the other lobe. Palpate both lobes while asking the patient to swallow.
10. Test for proximal myopathy. Ask the patient to rise from sitting without using their hands. Patients with hypothyroidism often can not manage this.
11. Test the knee jerk reflex. Patients who have hypothyroidism often have slow reflexes.
12. Thank the patient.

Exam favourites
- What are the clinical features of hypothyroidism?

Answer: overweight, peaches and cream complexion, cold hands, bradycardia, proximal myopathy, slow relaxing reflexes

- What are the three signs unique to Graves' disease?

Answer: pretibial myxoedema, thyroid acropachy and ophthalmoplegia.

13
Bone Disease and Parathyroids

Calcium homeostasis

In the UK, most people take between 0.5 g and 1 g of elemental calcium a day – mainly from dairy produce. Between 0.1 g and 0.7 g of calcium is excreted in urine and faeces. During growth there is increased intake (eg milk feeding in infants), increased absorption and decreased excretion. In the elderly, calcium intake tends to fall as does absorption, so there is a potential for calcium deficiency.

Serum calcium concentrations are regulated by parathyroid hormone (PTH), which is secreted by the four parathyroid glands. Low serum calcium stimulates PTH secretion. PTH increases serum calcium by:

- increase in selective tubular reabsorption of calcium
- increased production of 1,25 dihydroxyvitamin D, by increasing 1-hydroxylation of 25 OHD. I,25 OHD enhances calcium absorption from the gut.
- PTH enhances calcium release from the bones.

Hypercalcaemia

A raised serum calcium level may be artefactual due to prolonged stasis at venesection. True hypercalcaemia occurs in primary hyperparathyroidism, hypercalcaemia of malignancy and sarcoid. A large number of other causes are recognised but they are rare.

Hypercalcaemia may cause weakness, dizziness, anorexia, nausea, abdominal pain (peptic ulcer, renal stones) and mood swings. More severe cases present with polyuria, polydipsia, dehydration, confusion and coma.

Primary hyperparathyroidism

This causes hypercalcaemia due to excess PTH. This usually arises from a benign adenoma of one of the parathyroid glands although more than one gland may be affected (eg hyperplasia of all four glands). Malignancy of the parathyroids is rare. There is an association with previous neck irradiation and in 5% of cases primary hyperparathyroidism is part of a familial multiple endocrine neoplasia syndrome. Biochemically there is a high serum calcium with a non-suppressed PTH. X-rays may be normal or show a variety of features including nephrocalcinosis, subperiosteal resorption of the tufts of distal phalanges or distal clavicular osteopaenia. Osteitis fibrosa cystica is a feature of severe primary hyperparathyroidism and is characterised by cystic radiolucent areas, osteosclerosis and chondrocalcinosis.

Acute hypercalcaemia is treated by rehydration. Definitive treatment is surgical.

'Bones, stones, abdo groans and psychic moans' – think hyperparathyroidism

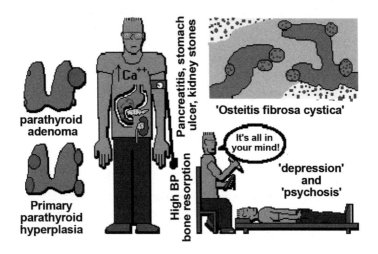

Figure 13.1 Primary hyperparathyroidism. Easy to diagnose and treat – if you think of it.

Hypercalcaemia of malignancy

Hypercalcaemia is a common feature of malignancy. It may result from multiple bony metastases but more usually is the result of production of PTH-related peptide (PTHrP) by the tumour. It is a feature of lung cancer, breast cancer, renal cancer and multiple myeloma. Initial treatment is rehydration; subsequently may be treated with bisphosphonates which bind to bone matrix and block osteoclastic bone resorption.

Sarcoidosis

Sarcoidosis is a chronic disease characterised by the formation of giant cell granulomas. These granulomas have the ability of hydroxylating 25 OHD to its active form 1,25 OHD, leading to hypercalcaemia.

Hypocalcaemia

A low serum calcium level may be artefactual if the serum albumin is also low. Causes of true hypocalcaemia include hypoparathyroidism, chronic renal failure, malabsorption and acute pancreatitis. A large number of other causes have also been described.

Clinically hypocalcaemia presents with paraesthesia, muscle cramps, tetany, carpopedal spasm, convulsions, alopecia and mucocutaneous candidiasis. Clinical signs include Chvostek's sign (tap on facial nerve) and Trousseau's sign (pump blood pressure cuff above systolic). Patients may also have dry skin, brittle nails and enamel hypoplasia.

Severe hypocalcaemia is usually seen in hypoparathyroidism due to autoimmune destruction or following neck surgery. Acute treatment is with intravenous calcium. Long-term treatment is with oral calcium (up to 2 g day) with or without vitamin D preparations.

Rickets and osteomalacia

Rickets (Figure 13.2) and osteomalacia are skeletal abnormalities that are caused by lack of calcium or phosphorous, but mainly due to lack of calcium absorption resulting from a diet deficient in vitamin D. Other causes include malabsorption and various vitamin D resistant states (eg inherited abnormalities of vitamin D receptor).

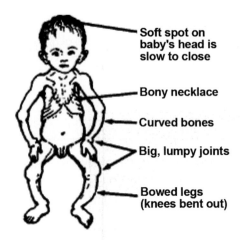

Figure 13.2 Signs of rickets.

In growing children, rickets results from deformities of the growing plates of bones and delayed/poor mineralisation. In adults, osteomalacia presents with bone pain but also muscle pain and weakness. Biochemically, calcium levels are low or normal and serum phosphate and vitamin D levels are low. PTH levels are high (secondary to low vitamin D and calcium) and alkaline phosphatase levels will also be high. Treatment is with vitamin D. Careful follow-up is required as it is possible to render patients hypercalcaemic with over-treatment using the currently available powerful vitamin D drugs.

Osteoporosis

Osteoporosis is loss of bone density (mineral and osteoid). It is a feature of ageing, particularly in post-menopausal women. Its development may be slowed by adequate dietary intake of calcium, alendronate, exercise and hormone replacement therapy.

Paget's disease

Paget's disease is a relatively common disease in which there is disordered bone turnover. Patients develop painful bones which become altered in shape, eg frontal bossing of the skull and bowing of the tibia.

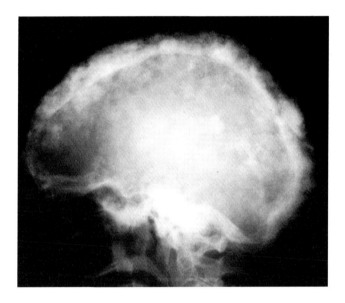

Figure 13.3 Typical radiographic appearance of the skull in Paget's disease.

14

Arthritis and Connective Tissue Disease

Osteoarthritis

Osteoarthritis is the term applied to 'wear and tear' arthritis. It increases in prevalence with age and results in considerable morbidity among the elderly. Premature osteoarthritis may occur if the joints have been placed under abnormal stress, eg deformities, obesity, athletes. Typically affects hips and knees but can affect any joint (Figure 14.1). Cervical spondylosis results from osteoarthritis of the many joints in cervical vertebrae and may lead to neck stiffness and reduced mobility. Compression of cervical nerve roots can lead to neurological symptoms in upper limbs. Symptoms are usually worse on exertion and relieved by rest. The classic physical sign is 'Heberden's nodes' on terminal interphalangeal joints. X-rays may show narrowing of joint space due to cartilage damage. Treatment is with analgesics, and obese patients should lose weight; severely affected joints may be replaced (eg hip replacement).

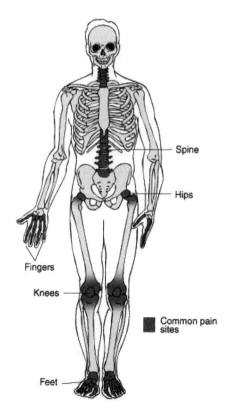

Figure 14.1 Common pain sites in osteoarthritis.

Spine

Hips

Fingers

Knees

Common pain sites

Feet

Rheumatoid arthritis

Rheumatoid arthritis is an immunologically mediated multisystem disease which has a particular proclivity for joints. It produces an erosive symmetrical small joint polyarthropathy characterised by synovial thickening. During an acute attack the joints are hot, swollen and extremely tender. Typical deformities arise including ulnar deviation of the fingers, z-thumb and swan-neck deformity of the interphalangeal joints (Figure 14.2). Chronic disease produces disorganised joints that are stiff but can improve with mobility. Extra-articular manifestations vary, including skin nodules, iritis, pulmonary nodules, fibrosis and pleural effusions, anaemia, splenomegaly. Some patients develop keratoconjunctivitis sicca (dry eyes). Treatment is initially with non-steroidal anti-inflammatory agents but penicillamine, gold or steroids may be needed.

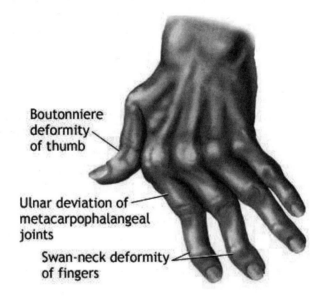

Boutonniere deformity of thumb

Ulnar deviation of metacarpophalangeal joints

Swan-neck deformity of fingers

Figure 14.2 Rheumatoid arthritis (late stage).

Eighty per cent of patients have IgM antibodies in their circulation, termed 'rheumatoid factor'. A variety of seronegative (ie no rheumatoid factor) arthritides are recognised. These include juvenile arthritis (Still's disease), ankylosing spondylitis, psoriatic arthropathy and Reiter's syndrome (urethritis, conjunctivitis and arthritis).

Gout

Gout is due to deposition of urate crystals in a joint. It typically affects the great toe but any joint may be affected. Serum uric acid levels are usually raised. Attacks may be precipitated by dehydration or use of drugs which reduce renal clearance of uric acid. Patients present with systemic upset and a hot, painful and swollen joint. Acute treatment is with colchicines, and chronic treatment is with allopurinol, which reduces plasma uric acid levels.

Systemic vasculitides (collagen vascular disease)

There are a number of poorly understood disorders characterised by inflammation of small arteries. They may present with rash, arthritis or renal failure.

Polymyalgia rheumatica and temporal arteritis

Polymyalgia rheumatica and temporal arteritis are disorders of middle/old age and may coexist. In polymyalgia, patients often present acutely with malaise, fever and pain/stiffness in the shoulder and/or pelvic girdle muscles. In temporal arthritis there may be a headache (unilateral, throbbing), scalp tenderness and jaw claudication (pain in the jaw brought on by prolonged chewing). The erythrocyte sedimentation rate (ESR) is high and temporal artery biopsy may reveal a giant cell vasculitis. Treatment is with high dose oral steroids to prevent optic nerve infarction and blindness.

Sjogren's syndrome

Affected people have dry eyes and mouth (although nose, throat, bronchi and vagina may be also affected). Many patients also have rheumatoid arthritis but it may occur as an isolated disorder. The parotid glands may be swollen and there is an increased incidence of dental caries.

Systemic lupus erythematosus (SLE)

SLE is more common in African Caribbeans and in women compared with men. Seventy per cent have a circulating antibody directed against double-stranded DNA. Certain drugs can cause lupus-like illness. Clinical features include:

- rash (usually in sun-exposed areas (eg butterfly rash))
- alopecia
- periungual infarcts
- cardiac involvement
- lung involvement
- nephritis
- neurological complications
- non-erosive arthropathy
- thrombotic tendency.

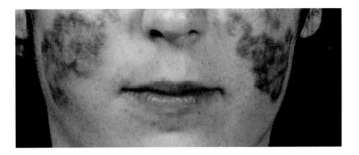

Figure 14.3 Classic butterfly rash.

Systemic sclerosis (scleroderma)

In this condition there is a progressive fibrosis and atrophy of the skin. A limited form of the condition is termed the CREST syndrome (calcinosis, Raynaud's phenomenon, oesophageal involvement, sclerodactyly and telangiectasia). A more widespread form may present with rapidly progressive hypertension and renal failure.

Other collagen vascular diseases include polyarteritis nodosa, polymyositis, dermatomyositis and Wegener's granulomatosis. Some of these patients are treated with high-dose oral corticosteroids which must not be stopped suddenly.

15
Renal Disease

Acute renal failure

Acute renal failure is a rapid severe decline in renal function. Although many patients have oliguria (< 500 ml urine/24 hours) some continue to pass reasonable volumes of urine, although the kidneys have lost the ability to concentrate toxic waste products in urine. Acute renal failure is divided into pre-renal, renal and post-renal failure.

Pre-renal failure

Pre-renal failure occurs when there is insufficient blood being delivered to the kidneys, eg hypovolaemia after a large haemorrhage, low cardiac output after a myocardial infarct or sepsis. In the early stages pre-renal failure may be reversed by improving renal perfusion – untreated intrinsic renal failure develops.

Intrinsic renal failure

Intrinsic renal failure is caused by a defect within the kidneys themselves. Apart from pre-renal failure, other causes include nephrotoxic drugs, haemolysis, rhabdomyolysis, malignant hypertension and glomerulonephritis.

Post-renal failure

The kidneys may fail if the outflow of urine is blocked, eg acute retention of urine following urethral trauma.

Patients in acute renal failure present in very varied ways. They may be dehydrated (pre-renal) or fluid overloaded (renal), and there may be signs of underlying sepsis, heart failure or multisystem disease.

Chronic renal failure

Chronic renal failure is a gradual decline in renal function. Renal function may be much impaired before there is any alteration in the serum urea and creatinine levels, but once these start to rise, the rise is often exponential. Renal function may be assessed by estimating the creatinine clearance or glomerular filtration rate (GFR). Patients with chronic renal failure may present with rapidly declining function (acute-on-chronic renal failure) due to one of the causes outlined above. Causes of chronic renal failure include chronic glomerulonephritis, diabetes, interstitial nephritis, renal vascular disease, multisystem diseases.

Patients present with many symptoms and signs including anaemia, nausea and vomiting, pruritus, pericarditis, metabolic acidosis and renal bone disease. End-stage renal failure is treated with dialysis (haemo- or peritoneal) or renal transplantation. However, decline in renal function can be slowed with careful management of hypertension, dehydration, urinary tract infection or obstruction and avoidance of nephrotoxic drugs. Vascular access is important in patients with renal disease – preserve all veins.

Acute nephritic syndrome

This is characterised by: haematuria, proteinuria, reduced renal function and salt and water retention. It used to be seen fairly commonly as a sequel to streptococcal infections. It also occurs in patients with some forms of glomerulonephritis.

Nephrotic syndrome

Nephrotic syndrome is characterised by heavy proteinuria resulting in hypoalbuminaemia and oedema. Causes include glomerulonephritis, diabetes, multisystem disease and certain drugs such as gold, penicillamine and captopril. Treatment involves fluid and salt restriction and a high-protein diet.

Glomerulonephritis

These are a group of disorders which may present with acute renal failure, chronic renal failure, nephritis or the nephrotic syndrome. They are classified according to histological features:

- minimal change glomerulonephritis – most common cause of childhood nephrotic syndrome
- focal and segmental glomerulosclerosis

- membranous glomerulonephritis – most common cause of adult nephrotic syndrome
- mesangiocapillary glomerulonephritis
- mesangial proliferative glomerulonephritis

Steroids and immunosuppressive agents are used in the treatment of these conditions.

Urinary tract infections

Urine is normally sterile. A urine sample may grow a mixture of organisms if it has been contaminated, either when it was taken or on its way to the laboratory. A heavy growth of organisms in a well-taken mid-stream urine (MSU) sample suggests significant infection. Urinary tract infections are more common in women, the elderly, catheterised patients, pregnant women and in those with congenital abnormalities of the urinary tract. Symptoms include polyuria and dysuria. Ascending infection may result in pyelonephritis. Common organisms include *Escherichia coli*, *Klebsiella* and *Proteus*. Treatment is with a course of oral antibiotics (eg trimethoprim, amoxicillin or ciprofloxacin). Recurrent infections require investigation. Symptoms of urinary tract infection with sterile MSU may be due to 'urethral syndrome'.

Renal stones

Stones may form in the kidney and then pass down the ureters. Stone formation is more common in patients with hypercalcaemia but may occur in otherwise healthy patients. Passing a renal stone causes intense pain in the loin, radiating to the groin and associated with dysuria and haematuria. The stone may become impacted in the ureter resulting in proximal hydronephrosis.

Renal tumours

Tumours may occur in the kidneys, bladder or prostate (rarely in ureters). They may present with a variety of features. In practice it is important to exclude neoplasia in all patients presenting with haematuria.

16
Anaemia and Bleeding Disorders

Normal physiology

Red cells are produced in the bone marrow from stem cells. The stimulus to red cell production is erythropoietin. This hormone is produced by the kidney in response to a number of stimuli including hypoxia and hypovolaemia. As the red cell matures, it accumulates haemoglobin and loses its nucleus. Iron is required for haemoglobin production. The rapid turnover of nuclear material in the dividing cells requires adequate B_{12} and folate stores. Anaemia means low haemoglobin (> 13.5 g/dl in men, and > 11.5 g/dl in women). It can be due to decreased production of red cells or increased loss (haemorrhage or haemolysis).

Clotting is mediated by a cascade of factors and the process can be divided into extrinsic (requires tissue factor for activation) and the intrinsic. In addition, functioning platelets are required. In practice, the most important aspect of first aid management of a bleeding patient is application of direct pressure to the site of bleeding or to the local arterial supply if it is accessible.

Symptoms of anaemia

Many patients have anaemia of gradual onset and present with non-specific symptoms, including tiredness and lethargy. Others may present with shortness of breath on exertion. Patients with impaired cardiac function may present in heart failure and anaemia can also precipitate worsening angina or peripheral vascular disease. Symptoms of the underlying condition causing anaemia may also be present, eg menorrhagia.

Signs of anaemia

Many patients with anaemia have no physical signs, whereas others look pale (examine the conjunctiva). However, most patients who look pale are not anaemic.

Acute haemorrhage

If patients bleed sufficiently, they will become anaemic. Haemoglobin measurement immediately after an acute bleed will be normal as there has been no time for haemodilution to occur; however a low Hb will be found the following day. Under normal situations with adequate iron, B_{12} and folate reserves, the anaemia is rapidly corrected by increased red cell production. Presence of reticulocytosis is a marker of this effect.

Chronic haemorrhage

Patients may become anaemic if they are slowly bleeding; this may be clinically inapparent. The slow bleeding results in iron deficiency. This is particularly the case in menstruating women and elderly people with poor diets. Menstruating women have poor iron reserves. Other causes include bleeding from peptic ulcers, oesophagitis and colonic lesions. Patients with telangiectasia in or around the mouth may have similar lesions in the bowel – hereditary haemorrhagic telangiectasia – and these may also bleed. Patients develop microcytic anaemia (low MCV) and also hypochromic red cells (low MCHC). Serum iron and ferritin levels will be low.

Every attempt should be made to find the source of bleeding since it may have a sinister cause. These patients are often investigated with endoscopy.

Treatment is with iron supplements. These can generally be given orally but sometimes need to be given parenterally.

Iron deficiency anaemia

This is usually due to chronic blood loss (see above). Sometimes it may occur without obvious blood loss – mainly in patients with poor dietary intake of iron.

B₁₂/folate deficiency

Apart from iron, B_{12} and folate are also required for the formation of red cells. Folate is absorbed in the proximal gut but B_{12} is absorbed in the terminal ileum attached to intrinsic factor, which is produced in the stomach. B_{12} and folate deficiency may occur due to dietary deficiencies. B_{12} deficiency occurs if there is failure of production of intrinsic factor (surgery or autoimmune disease). Small bowel disease such as Crohn's may lead to malabsorption of B_{12} and/or folate.

Patients develop macrocytic anaemia (raised MVC). In addition there is usually reduction in white cell count and platelets – pancytopenia. Bone marrow examination will show typical cells – the megaloblasts (premature red cells that have not developed properly due to lack of folate or B_{12}).

Folate may be replaced orally and is often combined with iron tablets (Fefol). Failure to absorb B_{12} is treated with parenteral B_{12}, usually in the form of monthly injections.

Other causes of macrocytosis include alcohol, liver disease and hypothyroidism.

Anaemia of chronic disease

Chronic diseases lead to anaemia. This may be a normochromic, normocytic anaemia with normal iron, B12 and folate levels. Patients in renal failure develop anaemia and this may be partly corrected by erythropoietin supplements.

Haemolytic anaemias

Anaemia may occur is red cells are prematurely destroyed in the circulation. This is termed haemolysis and may occur in a variety of infections. It also occurs when heart valves are abnormal. Certain inherited diseases such as thalassaemia, sickle cell disease and hereditary spherocytosis may lead to haemolytic anaemia.

Anaemia flow chart

The flow chart in Figure 16.1 shows an easy way to work out what sort of anaemia a patient has. Start by seeing if the patient has a macrocytic (raised MCV), microcytic (low MCV) or normocytic (normal MCV) anaemia and follow the flow chart.

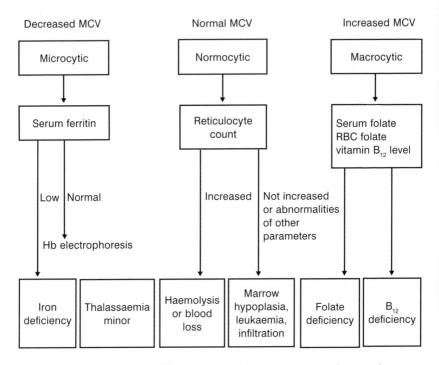

Figure 16.1 Flow chart to differentiate between the types of anaemia.

Transfusion

Blood transfusions are not without risk. There is the risk of fluid overload, transfusion reactions and spread of infections. Therefore transfusion should only be used in selected cases of anaemia – most cases can be dealt with by giving iron, B_{12} or folate supplements.

Bleeding disorders

Haemophilia a (factor VIII deficiency)

This is inherited as a sex-linked recessive condition. Often the family history is known or the condition is diagnosed in childhood following a haemarthrosis after a fall. Acure trauma causes bleeding which may appear to stop (due to action of platelet plug) – however, persistent oozing of blood then continues. Treatment is with factor VIII concentrate, which may be given prophylactically prior to procedures.

Haemophilia B (factor IX deficiency)

Haemophilia B presents like factor VIII deficiency but clearly needs factor IX concentrates. Clotting factors may be measured in a laboratory.

von Willebrand's disease

These patients have factor VIII deficiency but also a defect in platelet function. The condition can be quite mild.

Liver disease

The liver is the site of production of factors II, VII, IX and X and liver disease will cause decline in these to the extent of producing bleeding tendency. Always check coagulation profile (INR) in patients with suspected liver disease prior to surgery.

Anticoagulants

Most patients in dental practice who are taking anticoagulants will be taking oral warfarin. This causes a defect in the extrinsic coagulation pathway and thus mimics liver disease. Patients should have an international normalised ratio (INR) of between two to four times, normal depending on the indication for anticoagulation. Never stop warfarin without consulting a physician first. In some cases, eg recent pulmonary embolism, it is best to postpone dental treatment until after short-term coagulants are stopped. In other cases, it may be necessary to stop warfarin temporarily but cover patient with an intravenous infusion of heparin as an inpatient. Patients with artificial heart valves must never stop anticoagulation as the valve will thrombose, leading to death.

- Warfarin therapy may be reversed with vitamin K. However, this will make patients relatively resistant to warfarin for some days afterwards.
- Heparin is given intravenously or subcutaneously. It interferes with the intrinsic coagulation cascade and may be reversed with protamine.
- Tooth extraction is usually safe in patients on warfarin if the INR is < 3.5.

17
Headache and Cranial Nerve Defects

Headache is a common symptom and most patients do not have serious medical conditions; however, headache can be the presenting feature of a few severe illnesses and it is important to know in which cases the headache needs to be taken seriously.

Single episode of headache

After a head injury, headache is common. It usually resolves spontaneously and requires only simple analgesia unless the pain is particularly severe, there is drowsiness or vomiting or focal neurological signs develop.

Headache which is severe and of sudden onset with neck stiffness and perhaps focal neurological signs suggests the diagnosis of subarachnoid haemorrhage. These patients should be admitted to hospital urgently. Meningitis causes headache and neck stiffness. The headache is usually, but not always, severe. Systemic upset with fever is also present. Hangovers are a common cause of headache.

Recurrent attacks of headache

Recurrent attacks of headache are the feature of migraine. The cause of the attacks is thought to be decreased cerebral blood flow because of vasoconstriction. This is followed by vasodilatation, which gives the throbbing headache. Attacks may be preceded by visual aura. Headache often is unilateral. Often associated with nausea or vomiting. Attacks may be triggered by certain foods, chocolate, cheese or anxiety. Family history may be present. Photophobia is a feature and patients often prefer to sit quietly in the dark. Rarely associated with transient neurological deficit – hemiplegic migraine – but care should be taken in making this diagnosis. Cluster headaches are a type of migraine with recurrent unilateral headache associated with blood-shot and watering eye. These headaches are more common in men.

Treatment of the acute attack is with simple analgesics, together with antiemetics. A newer treatment is pizotifen which can be given as an injection or tablets. Frequent attacks may require prophylactic measures. These include β blockers and pizotifen.

Chronic headache

The most common cause is tension headache. The headache is often bilateral and feels like a pressure or weight on the area. It is present the whole day, often worsening in the evening. Raised intracranial pressure, eg from a brain tumour also produces a chronic headache. This headache is worse first thing in the morning, worse on bending or straining and may be associated with vomiting. Focal neurological deficits or blurring of vision may be present.

Temporal arteritis is a disease of middle/early aged patients with chronic headache or headache of sub-acute onset. Early diagnosis is vital as these patients are at risk of blindness from the associated optic nerve vasculitis. Treatment is with prompt high-dose steroids. The erythrocyte sedimentation rate (ESR) is much elevated and a temporal artery biopsy may show vasculitis.

Trigeminal neuralgia

Trigeminal neuralgia is a sharp stabbing pain along the distribution of the trigeminal nerve. It may be triggered by touching the face. Treatment is with phenytoin or carbamazepine.

Cranial nerve defects

I – Olfactory nerve
- Anosmia
- Common cold
- Fractures of cribriform plate
- Olfactory tract tumours
- Kalmann's syndrome

II – Optic nerve
- Decreased visual acuity
- Abnormal papillary reflexes
- Argyll Robertson pupil (small, irregular, reacts to accommodation but not light)
- Holmes–Adie pupil (delayed/absent response to light + accommodation, once constricted, dilates only slowly)

- Horner's syndrome (miosis, ptosis, anhidrosis, enophthalmos) – due to loss of sympathetic nerve fibres. Causes include:
    - Pancoast tumour
    - cervical rib
    - carotid aneurysm
    - syringomyelia
    - brain stem cardiovascular accident.

III – Oculomotor nerve

- Ptosis
- Pupil fixed and dilated
- Eyeball looks down and out.

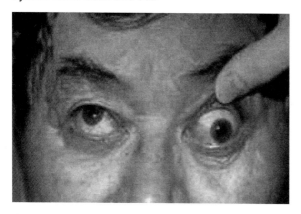

Figure 17.1 IInd nerve palsy: eyeball looks down and out.

IV – Trochlear nerve

- Impaired downward gaze with diplopia

V – Trigeminal nerve

- Motor loss – weakness of muscles of mastication
- Sensory loss – face, extent depends on which division of nerve is involved.

VI – Abducens nerve

Impaired lateral gaze with diplopia.

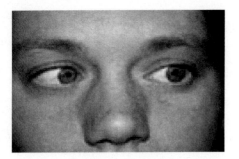

Figure 17.2 VIth nerve palsy.

VII – Facial nerve

- Paralysis of muscles of facial expression.
- Bell's palsy (Figure 17.3).
- Ramsay–Hunt syndrome due to herpes zoster infection of VII nerve – may have herpes vesicles in external auditory meatus or pharynx.

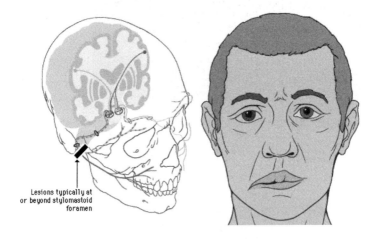

Lesions typically at or beyond stylomastoid foramen

Figure 17.3 Ipsilateral upper and lower facial asymmetry.

VIII – Vestibulocochlear nerve

- Deafness, tinnitus, vertigo.
- Acoustic neuromas.

IX – Glossopharyngeal nerve
• Sensation to posterior third of tongue, palate, pharynx.

X – Vagus nerve
• Motor supply to palate, pharynx, oesophagus.

XI – Accessory nerve
• Motor supply to larynx, pharynx, sternomastoid, trapezius.
• Recurrent laryngeal branch of vagus loops around aorta and runs a long course in neck – liable to damage in neck surgery.

XII – Hypoglossal nerve
• Motor supply to tongue and hyoid bone depressors.
• Lesions of the nerve cause unilateral paralysis, wasting and fasciculation of the tongue which is pushed over to the affected side when put out.

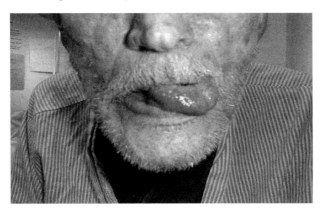

Figure 17.4 Hypoglossal nerve lesion.

Examination of the cranial nerves

I – Olfactory nerve
- Ask the patient if they have noticed any change in smell

II – Optic nerve
- Inspect the eye and note, pupil size, shape and equality
- Test for visual acuity
- Test for accommodation
- Test colour vision
- State that you would test the visual fields and perform funduscopy

III – Oculomotor nerve, IV – Trochlear nerve and VI – Abducens nerve
- Inspect the eyelid position for drooping
- Test the eye movements

V – Trigeminal nerve
- Check for sensation in the three divisions of the trigeminal nerve using a piece of cotton wool (Figure 17.5).

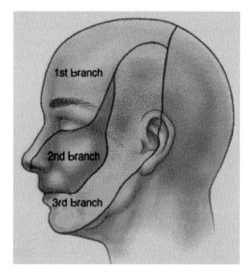

Figure 17.5 Distribution of the three divisions of the trigeminal nerve.

- Ask the patient to clench the muscles of mastication and check for
- Power in these.
- Test the jaw jerk reflex. Ask the patient to open their mouth. Rest your finger just below their lower lip and strike your finger gently with a patellar hammer

VII – Facial nerve

- Ask the patient to frown, close their eyes, blow their cheeks out and
- Show their teeth

VIII – Vestibulocochlear nerve

- Crudely examine the hearing by whispering in one ear and rustling a piece of paper in the other.

IX – Glossopharyngeal nerve; X – Vagus nerve

- Ask the patient to swallow and watch for nasal regurgitation.
- Look for a central uvula.
- Test the gag reflex with a tongue depressor.

XI – Accessory nerve

- Inspect the sternocleidomastoid and feel its bulk.
- Try and prevent the patient turning their head to one side and then repeat on the other side.
- Ask the patient to shrug their shoulders and try to resist them doing this.

XII – Hypoglossal nerve

- Ask the patient to stick their tongue out and look for deviation.
- Thank the patient.

18
Loss of Consciousness, Fits and Coma

There are many reasons for a loss of consciousness (LOC) or 'blackout'. First, it is important to understand what the patient means by a 'blackout'. Was the patient aware of:

- falling?
- of his or her surroundings?

What is the next thing he remembers. How long did the episode last? Has it occurred previously? The most common cause of LOC is probably the vaso-vagal attack or simple faint. This usually occurs with the patient upright. Many patients have had attacks previously and recognise the symptoms. Treatment is to return circulation to the brain by lying the patient down or having them put their head between their knees. Recurrent attacks merit some investigation.

Causes

Cardiac causes

LOC may occur if the cardiac output is suddenly impaired. This can occur due to cardiac arrhythmia, either bradycardia (eg heart block) or tachycardia. Such arrhythmias may occur in the face of an acute myocardial infarction or may represent disease of the conduction system per se. Treat by lying patient down in recovery the position. If there is no pulse, treat as cardiac arrest with cardiopulmonary resuscitation (CPR). Profound bradycardia requires iv atropine and perhaps insertion of a pacemaker. Ventricular fibrillation requires DC version.

Hypotensive causes

A sudden drop is blood pressure will cause blackout. This may occur during rapid haemorrhage (eg donating blood or gastrointestinal bleed). In the elderly or patients with steroid deficiency, postural hypotension occurs and LOC may occur on standing rapidly. This may also be a feature of young women especially when getting out of a hot bath.

Epilepsy

Care must always be taken in making the diagnosis of epilepsy as it has profound implications for employment, driving, insurance, etc. A single fit does not constitute epilepsy. The differential diagnosis includes syncope, pseudoseizures, hypoglycaemia, migraine and transient ischaemic attacks.

Epilepsy is broadly divided into a grand mal seizures (loss of consciousness, tonic-clonic jerks) and petit mal (may present with lack of attention, flicking eyelids – commoner in children). It may start with focal neurology, eg jerking of hand and then leads to LOC, jerking all limbs, urinary and faecal incontinence and tongue biting. Many cases are idiopathic. Family history is sometimes present. May follow head injury or be a feature of cerebrovascular disease. Can also occur as a result of metabolic derangements or hypoxia. Attacks in predisposed individual may be brought on by flashing lights, stress, tiredness, alcohol, some drugs. Aura may precede attack.

Treat by placing patient in recovery position. Move any objects likely to cause danger. Try to protect the airway (usually not possible) but make sure they are not left alone. If fit continues, use diazepam, iv or rectally. Check blood sugar to make sure patient is not hypoglycaemic – this is mandatory if there is any history of diabetes.

A first fit in middle age should always be investigated, including taking a computed tomography (CT) scan. The DVLA must be informed by patient of fits – driving may be permitted once the patient has been fit free for 2 years or having fits only at night. Patients may be permanently barred from certain occupations.

Long-term suppressive therapy is normally with anti-epileptics such as phenytoin and carbamazepine. These drugs should not be stopped. Certain other drugs will affect their metabolism and plasma levels, eg antibiotics. Phenytoin is associated with gingival hyperplasia but this can be reduced with good oral hygiene.

Other causes of LOC

These include drug misuse, alcohol intoxication and cough syncope.

Coma

This is a state of unawareness from which the patient cannot be roused. Sixty per cent of cases are due to metabolic derangement rather than primary neurological disease. The Glasgow Coma Scale (GCS) score gives as assessment of the depth of the coma by grading patients on eye movements, best verbal responses and best motor responses. It is imperative that all patients have a clear airway, which is protected until specialist help is available.

Brain tumours

About 30–40% of all brain tumours are metastases from elsewhere (eg lung, bowel) and herald the final stages of the disease. Intracranial metastases may be the presenting feature of cancer elsewhere.

Primary brain tumours need not be particularly malignant in that metastases outside the central nervous system are uncommon. However, they lead to problems because of raised intracranial pressure and neurological deficits. Tumours include gliomas and meningiomas. The prognosis with meningiomas is relatively good.

Patients may present with headache, visual disturbance, neurological deficits or fits. However, most patients with some or all of these symptoms do not have brain tumours. Investigations include computed tomography or magnetic resonance imaging, followed by stereotactic biopsy.

19
Neurological Disorders

Multiple sclerosis

This is a chronic disorder characterised by demyelination in the central nervous system. It affects about 1/2000 people in UK. An interesting aspect of its epidemiology is that the disease becomes increasingly common with increasing distance from the equator.

Multiple sclerosis often presents acutely with signs of a single area of demyelination (eg optic neuritis). Another attack may then not occur for many years (if at all). However, some patients have recurrent episodes of demyelination resulting in progressive disability. A few present a relentless progressive course. Symptoms and signs include vertigo, diplopia, nystagmus, cerebellar signs and progressive spastic paraparesis. Bladder and bowel function may be disturbed. Some patients show inappropriate euphoria but others are depressed. The diagnosis is made clinically aided by evidence of delayed visual evoked potentials, plaques on magnetic resonance imaging and raised levels of cerebrospinal fluid (CSF) protein with oligoclonal banding.

There is no specific treatment but high-dose intravenous steroids have been used in acute episodes. Recent trials have examined the possible benefit of interferon therapy. Patients benefit most from supportive care, including physiotherapy and counselling.

Parkinson's disease

Parkinson's disease is caused by progressive loss of neurones that radiate from the substantia nigra to the caudate nucleus and putamen in the mid-brain; these neurones use dopamine as a neurotransmitter. The typical clinical features are of rigidity (cog-wheel), bradykinesia and tremor (pin-rolling). Most are sporadic cases in the elderly but familial cases in younger patients are also recognised. As the disease progresses there is difficulty in maintaining balance, dysarthria and dysphonia, depression and dementia. Treatment includes dopamine agonists such as L-dopa and also selegiline.

Parkinsonism (as opposed to Parkinson's disease) may be because of other causes including:

- drugs – major tranquillisers such as the phenothiazines
- toxins – carbon monoxide
- Cerebrovascular disease
- Trauma, eg boxers.

Myasthenia gravis

Myasthenia gravis is an autoimmune disease where antibodies are present against muscle acetylcholine receptors. Patients develop increasing muscle weakness with prologues use of muscles and the disease presents with variable diploma, bulbar problems or weakness in the limb girdles (eg difficulty combing hair or climbing stairs). The muscle weakness may be exacerbated by pregnancy, and some drugs such as opiates and gentamicin. Diagnosis is with the Tensilon test (iv injection of an ultra-short-acting anticholinergic drug reverses the muscle weakness). Treatment is with longer acting anticholinergics such as neostigmine and pyridostigmine. Some cases are associated with a thymic tumour. Paradoxically, removal of the thymus in patients without a tumour often results in clinical improvement.

Motor neurone disease

In motor neurone disease there is progressive degeneration of anterior horn cells and cranial nerve nuclei. Patients present with upper and lower motor neurone signs but never any sensory loss. It is said that it never affects ocular movements. The disease pursues a relentless course with death within 5 years. Three different patterns of the disease are recognised:

- Progressive muscular atrophy – usually starts with wasting, weakness and fasciculation of the small muscles of the hands. Tends to spread proximally causing generalised upper limb weakness; a similar pattern occurs in the lower limbs.
- Amyotrophic lateral sclerosis – here there are signs of upper motor neurone degeneration (eg spasticity of the legs). Progressive muscular atrophy is also present so patients may have spastic lower limbs but flaccid upper limbs.

- Progressive bulbar palsy – patients present with dysarthria, dysphonia and difficulty in swallowing and chewing. The tongue is wasted and fasciculates. Paralysis of the respiratory muscles also occurs and death is usually due to aspiration pneumonia.

Disorders of peripheral nerves

Individual nerves may be affected by trauma or compression (eg median nerve at the wrist). When multiple individual nerves are affected the term 'mononeuritis multiplex' is used – causes include infarction of several nerves due to a systemic vasculitis or infiltration of several nerves by amyloid. The term polyneuropathy is applied when many peripheral nerves are affected – patients may present with numbness of the toes and fingers ('glove and stocking' distribution). There are a large number of disorders which may lead to polyneuropathy, such as:

- diabetes
- alcohol
- renal failure
- vitamin deficiency (B_{12})
- human immunodeficiency virus (HIV)
- drugs, eg phenytoin, lithium, gold
- systemic lupus erythematosus

20
Psychiatry for Dental Students

Organic brain syndromes

Patients with organic brain syndromes are not 'mentally ill' in the common sense of the term. They exhibit altered mental function as a result of an underlying medical condition. The most common form encountered is the acute toxic confusional state. Its features include:

- clouding of consciousness – this is important because patients with psychosis normally have clear consciousness
- disorientation
- visual hallucinations.

Common causes of an acute toxic confusional state include infection, drugs and dehydration. The term delirium tremens (DTs) is given to the specific acute confusional state that accompanies alcohol withdrawal. This may be seen in patients who are deprived of alcohol, eg in-patients, patients nil by mouth and patients in custody.

Chronic confusional states

The most common cause of chronic confusion is dementia. However, slowly progressive brain tumours, alcohol addiction, hypothyroidism and normal pressure hydrocephalus can all cause a similar clinical pattern. Patients often notice impairment of short-term memory but there is a global reduction in cognition and coarsening of the personality. The condition may occur in relatively young patients (pre-senile dementia). Alzheimer's disease is a specific pathological type of dementia, multi-infarct dementia being the other major type. All patients with dementia should be assessed by a doctor to exclude a treatable cause.

Depression

Everyone feels sad at some point or another. Depression is diagnosed when there are features suggestive of an abnormal mood. Reactive depression can be traced to a particular adverse life event. In some patients no trigger can be found – endogenous depression. Apart from 'feeling' sad, a variety of other symptoms are present, including:

- feelings of helplessness
- feelings of worthlessness
- early morning waking
- disturbed appetite
- negative views regarding future.

Most patients have depressive neurosis (insight preserved). Depressive psychosis is characterised by lack of insight and loss of contact with reality. Treatment is supportive, anti-depressants, psychotherapy or rarely electroconvulsive therapy (ECT).

Mania

Manic neurosis is not usually diagnosed since it may represent an ideal state of mind. Some patients develop euphoria and hyperactivity entirely out of proportion with normality. They lose insight and have manic psychosis. Often they speak rapidly and are full of grandiose ideas. They may feel they are very rich and enter into unwise financial situations. They sleep little, starting many projects but finishing very few. In many cases, the mania alternates with depression in bipolar affective disorder. Treatment is with lithium.

Schizophrenia

Schizophrenia is a specific diagnosis. While most people can 'understand' depression, mania, obsessions and phobias, schizophrenia appears totally removed from normal experience. Diagnosis is based on the presence of Schneider's 'first rank' symptoms, which include:

- thought insertion, broadcast or withdrawal
- auditory hallucinations in the third person
- passivity
- primary delusions.

These 'positive symptoms' eventually give way to 'negative symptoms' of extreme withdrawal and social isolation. Treatment is with major tranquillisers.

Paranoia

Paranoia is the feeling that 'someone is out to get me'. It can be a feature of schizophrenia and can also be seen in alcoholics and drug misusers.

Phobia

Phobias are irrational fears. Some have some basis in fact but the fear is disproportionate to the likely outcome. They are readily amenable to therapy. Treatment may be by gradual introduction of the feared situation or by the short-term use of anxiolytics.

Obsessional neurosis

Patients with this condition have recurrent ruminations which are upsetting but which they feel unable to control. Subjects often perform tasks repeatedly – compulsive disorder. Often co-exists with depression.

Anorexia/bulimia

Eating disorders are very common in young adults, especially women. Bulimia may result in dental erosion from repeated coating of teeth with gastric acid. Blistering of the knuckles can also be seen from recurrent self-induced vomiting.

Learning disability

It is important to distinguish this from mental illness. These patients have impaired mental function due to brain damage. A variety of syndromes of mental handicap exist. Many children with learning disabilities are bruxists.

21
Childhood Illnesses

Measles

Measles is a common and highly infectious viral illness. It can result in serious sequelae and consequently is the subject of a vaccination campaign. All children are offered measles vaccine as part of the MMR jab. The incubation period (ie time between infection with the virus and clinical features) is between 10 and 14 days. The child is infectious during this time after which he or she develops fever, cold-like symptoms and conjunctivitis. Koplik's spots are small white spots surrounded by erythema on the buccal mucosa. After 3–4 days a maculopapular rash appear usually head and neck and then spreads to rest of body. The ash may become blotchy, lasts for 3–4 days and then disappears as the child improves. Complications include bronchopneumonia, otitis media and rarely encephalitis.

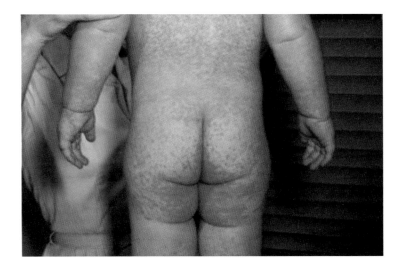

Figure 21.1 Measles.

Rubella (German measles)

Rubella is a mild disease. Incubation period is between 14 and 21 days followed by lymphadenopathy (especially suboccipital) and coryza and a pink macular rash. Main concern is the devastating effect of infection during pregnancy. In the UK, rubella antibody status is checked in all females in the ante-natal clinic. Vaccination is given as part of MMR.

Chicken pox

Chicken pox is also usually a mild disease in children although it can lead to more problems in adults. The cause is infection with the varicella zoster virus. The incubation period is around 2 weeks and child may be well, apart from a low-grade pyrexia. The spots appear in crops (Figure 21.2) progressing from macule to papule to vesicle. The vesicle dries and scabs and these fall off, generally without scarring unless secondary infection supervenes.

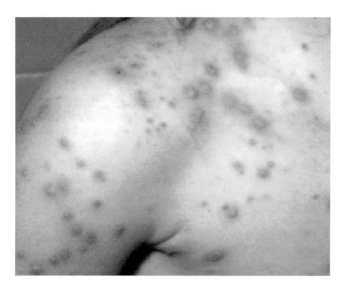

Figure 21.2 Chicken pox.

Lesions may also occur on the mucous membranes, especially in the mouth, where they rupture to produce shallow ulcers. Very rarely chicken pox can produce an encephalitis which presents with ataxia due to cerebellar involvement. Pneumonia may occur – but this is mainly in adults. Chicken pox can be very severe with a haemorrhagic rash in the immunosuppressed patient. Herpes zoster tends to erupt in a dermatomal pattern as seen in Figure 21.3. If it affects the face it can lead to the Ramsay–Hunt syndrome and deafness. Reactivation of the Herpes zoster infection is commonly known as shingles and is found in a dermatomal region. The most common dermatomal region is the maxillary division of the trigeminal nerve or some of the thoracic dermatomes.

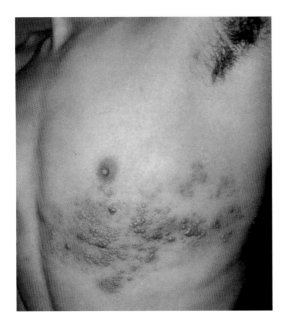

Figure 21.3 Herpes zoster.

Mumps

Mumps is caused by a paramyxovirus and subclinical infection is very common. The incubation period can be as long as 3 weeks, followed by fever and malaise and swelling of one or both parotid glands. The submandibular glands may also be affected. Mild viral meningitis may supervene. Patients complain of earache and difficulty swallowing. Epididymo-orchitis is a rare complication before puberty. Pancreatitis is a recognised but rare complication, and it must be distinguished from cervical lymphadenopathy.

Glandular fever

Glandular fever is most common in adolescence but can also occur in children. It is also termed infectious mononucleosis and is caused by the Ebstein–Barr virus. The disease is spread by close contact since the virus is present in nasopharyngeal secretions. Onset is usually insidious with an incubation period of 4–14 days. Patients may present with anorexia, malaise and fever and usually have a sore throat and enlarged glands. Petechiae may occur on the palate. Splenomegaly may occur and a rash – especially if ampicillin is given. Hepatitis with jaundice may occur. Pneumonitis is rare. The diagnosis is based on the finding of irregular monocytes on blood film. Horse red cells are agglutinated (monospot test) and antibodies can be detected (Paul Bunnell test). Lymphadenopathy and splenomegaly may persist for months associated with a long period of debility.

Scarlet fever

Scarlet fever s results from infection with a strain of group A haemolytic streptococci that produce an erythrogenic toxin. A short incubation period of 2–4 days is followed by tonsillitis, rash, fever and malaise. A fine punctuate erythematous rash develops, which blanches on pressure. The face spared but cheeks are flushed. The tongue develops a thick white coating through which the inflamed papillae project (white strawberry tongue). After 4–5 days, the tongue peels leaving a red strawberry appearance. Treatment with penicillin leads to rapid recovery. As the rash fades, there is desquamation on the hands and feet, which may allow a retrospective diagnosis.

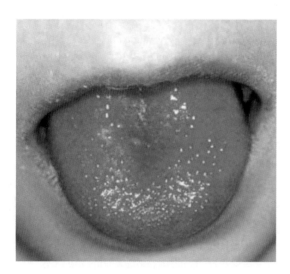

Figure 21.4 Scarlet fever – classic strawberry tongue.

Pertussis (whooping cough)

This is caused by *Bordetella pertussis* and is a prolonged respiratory illness. After a 7-day incubation period, there is a catarrhal stage of 1–2 weeks when the child is unwell with coryza. The child then has a paroxysmal whooping cough that can last 4–6 weeks and may lead to bronchopneumonia. Especially dangerous in infancy. Treatment is largely symptomatic, nursing care, suction, oxygen. Some give erythromycin but probably only helpful in early stages. No help once coughing spasms are established.

Infectious gastroenteritis

Many possible organisms are responsible. The most common cause are rotaviruses, which can spread rapidly within a community. May cause severe illness in the compromised and lead to serious disruption in institutions.

Prevention

Any child with rash should be seen by his or her general practitioner prior to attending school/parties, etc. Do not allow parents to bring children into your surgery for 48 hours after last bout of diarrhoea and vomiting if you wish to stop yourself, your staff and other patients catching the infection.

22

Dermatology

Psoriasis

Psoriasis is a common disease that can affect any age group. The rash is typically 'salmon pink' with silvery scales, affecting the extensor surfaces in a symmetrical pattern. Psoriasis in the flexures may not be scaly and other sites commonly affected are the scalp, umbilicus and peri-anal region. The nails may show pitting, onycholysis and thickening. Around 10% of patients develop an arthropathy that typically affects the distal interphalangeal joints and large joints such as the knees. It is a sero-negative erosive arthritis. Pustular psoriasis is rare but may occur on the palms and soles.

Treatment is with coal tar soaps, dithranol or psoralens, along with UV light.

Dermatitis

Dermatitis is inflammation of the skin; there are a number of common types:
- Atopic dermatitis = eczema:
  - usually begins in childhood
  - 70% have family history of atopy
  - > 90% resolve by teenage
  - flexures often affected and also knees, elbows, wrists, ankles
  - secondary infection may occur.
- Neurodermatitis: chronic dermatitis perpetuated by scratching.
- Chronic dermatitis: allergy to a variety of substances.
- Nickel, perfume, chemicals.
- Stasis dermatitis: seen around chronic venous ulcers in legs.
- Seborrhoeic dermatitis: cradle cap in infancy. There is scaling in the scalp and around the ears in adults.

Urticaria

This is the pruritic, erythematous swelling caused by fluid leaking from the blood vessels in the skin to the dermis. It may follow an insect sting, food allergy or drug hypersensitivity.

Skin tumours

A number of malignant and pre-malignant changes occur in the skin:

- Solar keratoses: occur on sun-exposed areas as a scaly erythematous patch.
- May become malignant after many years.
- Basal cell carcinoma: slow-growing, locally invasive malignant tumour (Figure 22.1). Begins as slowly enlarging nodule which then ulcerates to leave a shallow ulcer surrounded by a raised 'pearly' edge.
- Squamous cell carcinoma: occur in sun-exposed areas. Unlike basal cell carcinoma, squamous cell carcinomas tend to have thick edges and irregular bases (Figure 22.1).
- Secondary tumours: some primary cancers metastasise to skin, eg lung cancer.

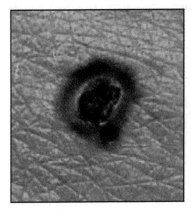 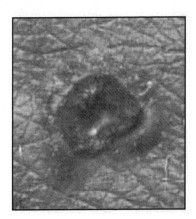

Figure 22.1 Squamous cell carcinoma (left) and basal cell carcinoma (right).

Malignant melanomas

Moles (congenital melanocytic naevi) appear during the first few years of life. Most people have < 40. Moles should be uniformly pigmented with a regular margin. If a pigmented lesion changes in size or colour, or itches and bleeds, it should be considered as potentially malignant (Figure 22.2).

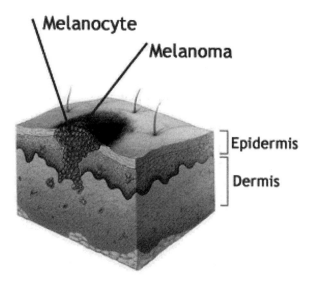

Figure 22.2 Melanoma.

Malignant melanomas may arise in pre-existing moles or may arise de novo. Sun exposure greatly increases the risk of developing malignant melanoma. A few melanomas are non-pigmented and are easy to miss. Melanoma may spread to the liver, lungs and brain as well as other distant sites.

Skin infections

- Bacterial:
    - staphylococcal (impetigo, furuncle, toxic epidermal necrolysis)
    - streptococcal (erysipelas)
    - tuberculosis
    - leprosy
    - syphilis.
- Viral:
    - human papilloma virus (warts)
    - herpes simplex I and II
    - herpes zoster (chickenpox, shingles)
    - Molluscum contagiosum (pox virus).

- Fungal:
    - 'ringworm'
    - athlete's foot
    - candidiasis.
- Infestations:
    - insect bites
    - scabies.

23
Oral Manifestations
of Medical Conditions

Gastroenterology

- Coeliac disease: glossitis, stomatitis, angular cheilitis, oral ulceration.
- Ulcerative colitis: aphthous ulcers, pyostomatitis vegetans.
- Crohn's disease: ulcers – gingival, buccal mucosa, lips, granulomatous cheilitis.
- Cirrhosis: glossitis
- Peutz–Jeghers syndrome: pigmented lesions.
- Gardeners' syndrome: sebaceous cysts.
- Hereditary haemorrhagic: telangiectasia

Haematology

- Anaemia: atrophic glossitis, angular cheilitis.
- Leukaemia: ulceration, haemorrhages.
- Myeloma: macroglossia.

Endocrinology

- Acromegaly: macroglossia, large lips, widely spaced teeth, mandible growth, malocclusion.
- Addison's disease: pigmentation.
- Cushing's syndrome: candidiasis.
- Hypothyroidism: macroglossia in congenital cases.
- Diabetes: dry mouth.

Neurology

- Trigeminal nerve:
    - motor root – muscles of mastication
    - sensory root – abnormal sensations in teeth, palate; taste not affected.
- Facial nerve:
    - motor root – muscles of facial expression
    - sensory root – taste to anterior two-thirds of tongue.
- Temporal arteritis: jaw claudication.
- Motor neurone disease: wasted, weak and fasciculating tongue.

Cardiovascular

- Angina: pain in jaw.

Respiratory

- Respiratory failure: central cyanosis.

Other diseases

- Malignancy: secondary deposits.
- Amyloid: macroglossia.
- Immunosuppressed: gingivitis, candidiasis.
- Lead poisoning: dark line at gingival margin.
- Behçet' s syndrome: oro-genital ulceration.
- Measles: Koplik's spots.
- Infectious mononucleosis: petechiae at junction of hard and soft palate.

24
Sexually Transmitted Diseases and AIDS

Human immunodeficiency virus (HIV) infection and Acquired immune deficiency syndrome (AIDS)

AIDS results from infection with HIV. HIV is a retrovirus which infects and destroys CD4 (helper) T lymphocytes. Most common type is HIV 1 although others are being recognised (eg HIV 2).

HIV virus has been found in blood, semen, vaginal secretions, tears and saliva. Infection through contact with tears and saliva is a theoretical possibility but has not been proved unequivocally. A few cases of HIV infection have been reported where oral contact was the only reported risk factor but these have been subject to debate. No cases of HIV infection have been reported among dentists or endoscopists where the only contact has been with saliva. The main occupational risk is from needle-stick injuries. A risk of acquiring HIV from a single needle-stick injury from an infected patient is probably < 1%, but depends on a number of factors including the size of the inoculum.

Major risk factor for HIV infection is receptive intercourse (anal or vaginal). Concurrent genital ulceration increases the risk. Risk assessment and management is a complex issue but the following points are worth bearing in mind:

- It is possible to be infected with HIV from a single needle-stick injury or sexual encounter. Even if the person involved does not appear to belong to a high risk group, it is usually not possible to be certain they are not affected. Thus it is sensible to behave as if all patients are potentially infected.
- HIV seropositive rates range from 1:5 among homosexuals attending genitourinary clinics in London to < 1:500 women attending ante-natal clinics. Since a single exposure to a known carrier will only result in sero-conversion in < 1% of cases, the risk of infection from a casual contact or injury is numerically small. The concerns arise because the risk is finite and infection has profound implications.

Practical points
- Always sterilise equipment between patients.
- Always wear gloves.
- Always disinfect/discard blood stained items.
- Learn how to dispose of needles properly.
- Always use approved clinical waste disposal systems.

If you have a needle-stick injury:

- Do not panic.
- Encourage free bleeding from the site.
- Is the patient known HIV positive? Does he or she belong to a high risk group? This information may help you feel better but, as discussed above, will not completely settle the issue.
- Explain to the patient what has happened.
- Seek the advice of an occupational health physician or HIV counsellor. If you wish, you may have an HIV test; however this will need to be performed twice. The first test will confirm whether or not you have previously been infected. If this is negative but a second test 3 months later is positive, there is evidence you have seroconverted as a result of the injury. You will have to avoid all other risk activity in the period of time between the two tests.
- You will need to consider how you would cope with a positive first or second test.
- Some insurance companies will offer cover against HIV infection contracted during your work. However, you will have to prove that the infection was directly attributable to your work by undergoing the two tests as described above.

Remember: you are more likely to contract hepatitis B than HIV and you should be vaccinated and have adequate protection against hepatitis B.

HIV testing

The test measures antibody levels. It may take 3 months (rarely longer) for seroconversion to occur so tests should be performed at least 3 months after all risk behaviour.

Clinical course

In the first few weeks/months, there may be an acute seroconversion illness. This may present with a sore throat, rash, fever, malaise. Rarely the seroconversion illness is severe with encephalitis. There then follows a variable but prolonged asymptomatic phase during which CD4 lymphocyte levels fall. The patient remains infective but there is evidence to suggest that infectivity increases as the patient progresses to full AIDS.

Patients may then present with persistent generalised lymphadenopathy, enlarged tonsils, weight loss, malaise. Progression occurs to AIDS-related complex (ARC). At this stage oral candidiasis, hairy leukoplakia, herpes simplex or zoster may become apparent and patients continue to lose weight and develop a pancytopenia.

AIDS is diagnosed when an HIV-positive patient develops a major opportunistic infection or some malignancies (eg Kaposi's sarcoma) for which no other cause can be found, such as:

* *Pneumocystis carinii* pneumonia (PCP)
* cytomegalovirus pneumonia, retinopathy, encephalitis
* cryptococcal brain abscess
* severe herpes zoster/simplex.

Patients may also develop resistant diarrhoea, lymphomas and dementia.

Treatment

A number of antivirals have been tried in HIV-positive patients in an attempt to delay or prevent the progression to AIDS. Prophylaxis against PCP is also used. Opportunistic infections are treated with high-dose antibiotics/antivirals or antifungal agents as required.

Other sexually transmitted diseases

Sexually transmitted diseases may affect the oral cavity either by direct sexual contact or as part of the systemic manifestations of some of the infections:

* Gonococcal pharyngitis
* Syphilis
    - primary chancre
    - snail track ulcers
    - gumma.
* Herpes simplex.

25
Clinical Genetics

Definitions

Monogenic disease

This is a disease due to a defect in a single gene. Examples include cystic fibrosis, alpha$_1$-antitrypsin deficiency, tuberculous sclerosis.

Polygenic disease

Genetic factors play a part in the development of many diseases, eg diabetes, heart disease, dementia. However, there is increased risk because of multiple genes acting in synergy. Environmental factors play an important part in modifying the expression of polygenic disorders. Thus an individual may have inherited several genes contributing to hypertension, but the disorder may not become manifest unless the patient has a diet high in salt or becomes obese.

Autosomal dominant disease

Autosomal dominant disease is a monogenic disorder in which a single abnormal gene is sufficient to cause clinically overt disease. Examples include achondroplasia, Marfan's syndrome and neurofibromatosis. Typically, one parent is affected and will pass on the disease to 50% of the offspring.

Autosomal recessive disease

Autosomal recessive disease is a monogenic disorder in which the disease is only manifest when a person inherits two abnormal genes (homozygous). Examples include cystic fibrosis, thalassaemia and congenital adrenal hyperplasia. Typically neither parent is clinically affected but they both carry one copy (heterozygote) of the abnormal gene and 25% of offspring are affected.

Sex-linked disorders

Abnormalities on the Y chromosome will only ever affect males. X chromosome abnormalities usually only affect males since most are recessive and females will usually have a normal X chromosome as well as the defective copy.

Chromosomal abnormalities

These include Down's syndrome (trisomy 21), Edwards' syndrome (trisomy 18), Turner's syndrome (XO) and Klinefelter's syndrome (XXY).

Genetic counselling

Parents are often concerned about the risk of passing diseases onto their children, especially if a disorder is known to run in the family. Previously it was only possible to give broad risks, eg 50% chance for autosomal dominant, 25% chance for recessive, etc. Increasingly the specific gene defects responsible for diseases are being discovered. It therefore becomes possible to give more accurate information to parents regarding risk. This major medical advance has also brought important ethical considerations. Thus it would be possible to test you for carriage of the various mutations associated with cystic fibrosis. If you knew you were carrying a defect it might have important implications regarding whether you chose a spouse who also knew he or she carried the gene defect. It is possible to test for affection status pre-term and this has led to selective abortion of affected fetuses.

Acquired and somatic mutations

Apart from inherited, germ-line gene defects, mutations also occur in DNA throughout life. If a mutation occurs in a key regulatory gene (eg an oncogene), the affected cell may start to proliferate and this underlies a number of malignancies. The malignant potential of radiation and certain drugs is related to their ability to produce DNA mutations.

26

Examination of the Acutely Unwell Patient

When examining an unwell patient it is always very important to have a systematic approach to the patient. You should always approach the patient from an ABDCEFGHI perspective:

A – Airway, B – Breathing, C – Circulation, D – Disability, E – Exposure, F – Fluid balance, G – Gas (Arterial blood gas), H – Hb (blood test results), I – Impression.

A – airway

Talk to the patient. Is the patient able to talk in sentences? If the patient is able to talk clearly to you then the airway is likely to be clear. Listen to hear if there are any noises such as stridor (inspiratory wheeze) which may indicate a foreign body in the airway.

B – breathing

- What is the respiratory rate (normal 12–16)?
- What is the chest expansion like?
- Is the chest expanding equally?
- Is the patient taking deep or shallow breaths?
- Is there air entry in all zones of the lungs?
- Are there any crackles or wheezes?
- If there are wheezes, is it an inspiratory wheeze or an expiratory wheeze?
- Is the trachea centrally placed?
- What are the oxygen saturations?

C – circulation

- Is the patient warm in the periphery?
- What is the heart rate?
- Are pulses present peripherally?
- Is the pulse regular, regularly irregular or irregularly irregular?
- What is the blood pressure?
- Are there any added heart sounds (murmurs)?
- Is there any ankle oedema?

D – disability

- What is the Glasgow Coma Scale (GCS) or AVPU (Alert, responds to Voice, responds to Pain, Unresponsive) score?
- What is the blood sugar level of the patient – this will help rule out hyper- and hypoglycaemia.
- Is the patient confused?
- If so are they normally confused?
- Has the patient started any medications or opiates recently?

E – exposure

- Is the abdomen soft and non-tender?
- Are any organs palpable?
- Is there any obvious signs of trauma?
- Is there anything abnormal about the patient?
- Has the patient opened their bowels recently?

F – fluid balance

- What is the urine output of the patient? (A patient should pass around 30 ml of urine per hour as a rough guideline.)
- How much fluid has the patient had within the past 24 hours? (A patient should normally have 3 litres of fluid per day.)

G – arterial blood gas

This is a very valuable test that gives you rapid blood results for a patient. It will quickly tell you the haemoglobin, lactate, pO_2, pCO_2, sodium, potassium, calcium, chloride, and pH. This will give you an insight into how unwell the patient is and any obvious causes.

H – haemoglobin (normal bloods)

It is important to check the results of any blood tests which have been done recently, and to take a new set of blood samples as well.

I – impression

From all the above information, you must form an impression for the cause of the unwell patient and then order tests which you feel will assist making a diagnosis for the patient. It is also important to gain iv access for the patient to begin treating them.

Index

ABCDE examination 175–6
abdominal examination 60
abducens nerve 123–4, 126
accessory nerve 125, 127
acute coronary syndromes (ACS) 10,
  12–15
Addison's disease 88
adrenal gland 87–9
adrenocorticotropic hormone (ACTH) 80,
  81, 87
AIDS 52, 165–7
alcohol withdrawal 141
aldosterone 88
allergies 4, 45, 47, 58, 155
amyotrophic lateral sclerosis 136
anaemia 113–16
anaesthesia 44, 51, 73
androgens 89
angina 10–11, 162
angiography 11
angioplasty 11, 14
antibiotics 26, 51, 52
anticoagulants 15, 35, 118
antidiuretic hormone (ADH) 80
aortic valve 21, 22
arrhythmia, cardiac 18, 37, 130
arteriosclerosis 9–15, 75, 162
arteritis 103, 122
arthritis 101–3
asbestos 47, 54
ascites 64
asthma 45–7
atherosclerosis 9–15, 75, 162
atrial fibrillation 18, 37
auscultation 16–17, 21–2, 39

basal cell carcinoma 156

beta blockers 10, 15
biliary disease 68
bipolar affective disorder 142
blood clotting see clotting
blood glucose in diabetes 71, 72–3, 74,
  76
blood loss 57, 113, 114
blood pressure 29, 30–1, 130
blood transfusion 116
bone disease 93–7
bowel disease 58–60
brain tumours 132
bronchial carcinoma 54
bronchitis 43–4
bruxism 143
bulimia 143

calcium 93–5
calculi, renal 109
cancer
  aetiology 172
  brain 132
  colon 59
  hypercalcaemia and 93, 94
  kidney 109
  pituitary 79
  respiratory system 54
  skin 156–7
  thyroid 87
cardiovascular system
  anatomy and physiology 9, 21, 29
  arrhythmia 18, 37, 130
  atheromatous disease 9–15, 75, 162
  congenital disease 26
  examination 5, 15–18, 175
  heart failure 29–30
  valvular disease 21–6

chest pain 10, 12
chicken pox 148
childhood disease 53, 85, 95–6, 147–51
chronic obstructive pulmonary disease
    (COPD) 43–5
clotting 113
    anticoagulants 15, 35, 118
    bleeding disorders 63, 117
clubbing, of digits 16
coagulation see clotting
coeliac disease 58
collagen vascular diseases 103–4, 122
colon 59–60
coma 132
confusional states 141
Conn's syndrome 88
consciousness
    clouded 64, 141
    loss of 130–2
coronary arteries 9, 10, 11
cortisol 87–8
counselling, genetic 172
cranial nerves 122–7, 161
Crohn's disease 58
CURB 65 (pneumonia) 53
Cushing's syndrome 80, 87–8
cystic fibrosis 53, 172

deep vein thrombosis (DVT) 35, 36
delirium 141
dementia 141
depression 141–2
dermatitis 155
dermatology see entries at skin
diabetes mellitus 71–6
diverticular disease 60
Duke's criteria 25–6
duodenal ulcers 57–8
dysphagia 57

eating disorders 143
eczema 155

electrocardiograms (ECGs) 12–13,
    17–18
emphysema 44–5
encephalopathy, hepatic 64
endocarditis 24–6
endocrinology 79–81, 85–9, 161
epilepsy 131
examination see physical examination
exercise testing 11
extrinsic allergic alveolitis 47
eye, signs of disease 38, 75, 79, 86,
    122–3

face, signs of disease 16, 38
facial nerve 124, 127, 161
fainting 130
family history 4
fibrosis, pulmonary 47
fits 131
fluid balance 71–2, 176
folate 115
follicle-stimulating hormone (FSH) 80, 81
foreign body inhalation 48

gastroenteritis 151
gastrointestinal system 5, 57–60, 161
gastro-oesophageal reflux disease 57
genetics 4, 171–2
German measles 147
glandular fever 149–50
glomerulonephritis 108–9
glossopharyngeal nerve 125, 127
glucocorticoids 87–8
glucose, blood levels 71, 72–3, 74, 76
gluten enteropathy 58
gout 103
Graves' disease 86–7, 89
growth hormone 80, 81

haematemesis 57
haematology
    anaemia 113–16

coagulopathy 63, 117
oral signs of disease 161
haemolytic anaemia 115
haemophilia 117
haemorrhage 57, 113, 114
hand
  arthritis 102
  signs of disease 16, 38
headache 121–2
heart *see* cardiovascular system
Heimlich's manoeuvre 48
Helicobacter pylori 57
heparin 35, 118
hepatic disease 63–8, 117, 166
hepatitis, viral 66–7, 166
history taking 3–5
hormonal disorders 79–81, 85–9, 161
Horner's syndrome 38, 123
human immunodeficiency virus (HIV) 52,
  165–7
hypercalcaemia 93–5
hyperprolactinaemia 79–80
hypertension
  portal 64
  systemic 30–1
hyperthyroidism 86–7, 89
hypocalcaemia 95
hypoglossal nerve 125, 127
hypoglycaemia 73, 76
hypotension 130
hypothyroidism 85–6, 89

immunosuppressed patients 52,
  165–7
infectious mononucleosis 149–50
infective endocarditis 24–6
inflammatory bowel disease 58–9
insulin therapy 72, 73
international normalised ratio (INR) 118
iron 114
irritable bowel syndrome 59–60

jaundice 63, 68
Jones's criteria 23–4

kidney disease *see* renal disease

large bowel 59–60
learning disability 143
liver disease 63–8, 117, 166
liver function tests 65
loss of consciousness (LOC) 130–2
lung anatomy and physiology 43
lung disease 43–8, 51–4, 151
lung function tests 40, 45
luteinising hormone (LH) 80, 81

malabsorption 58
malignant hypertension 31
mania 142
mean cell volume (MCV) 116
measles 147
medical history 4
melanoma 156–7
meningitis 121
mental illness 141–3
mesothelioma 54
migraine 121
mineralocorticoids 88
mitral valve 21, 22
motor neurone disease 136–7
mouth, signs of medical conditions
  161–2
multiple sclerosis 135
mumps 149
myasthenia gravis 136
myocardial infarction 12–15, 75

needle-stick injuries 165, 166
nephritic syndrome 108–9
nephrotic syndrome 108
neuropathy 135–7, 161
  cranial nerves 122–7, 161
  diabetic 75–6

nosocomial pneumonia 51–2

obsessional neurosis 143
oculomotor nerve 123, 126
oesophagus 57
olfactory nerve 122, 126
optic nerve 122–3, 126
oral hypoglycaemic drugs 74
oral signs of medical conditions 161–2
organic brain syndromes 141
osteoarthritis 101
osteomalacia 95–6
osteoporosis 96
ovary 81
oxygen therapy 43, 44

pacemakers 37
paediatric disease 53, 85, 95–6, 147–51
Paget's disease 97
pain, history of 3
paranoia 143
parathyroid hormone (PTH) 93–4
parkinsonism 136
Parkinson's disease 135
peak expiratory flow measurement
   (PEFR) 40
peptic ulcers 57–8
percussion, chest 39
peripheral neuropathic disease 76, 137
peripheral vascular disease 15, 35
pernicious anaemia (B_{12} deficiency) 115
pertussis 151
phenytoin 131
phobia 143
physical examination 5–6
   abdominal 60
   acutely unwell patients 175–6
   cardiovascular 5, 15–18, 175
   cranial nerves 126–7
   respiratory 5, 38–40, 175
   thyroid 89
pituitary gland 79–81

platelets 64, 117
pleural cancer 54
pneumoconiosis 47
pneumonia 51–2
polymyalgia rheumatica 103
polyneuropathy 76, 137
portal hypertension 64
progressive bulbar palsy 137
progressive muscular atrophy 136
prolactin 79–80
psoriasis 155
psychiatric disorders 141–3
psychosis 142–3
pulmonary embolism 36–7
pulmonary fibrosis 47
pulmonary valve 21, 22

rashes 104, 155
   paediatric 147, 148, 150
red blood cells 113
renal disease 15, 109
   diabetic 75
   nephritic syndrome 108–9
   renal failure 107–8, 115
respiratory system
   anatomy and physiology 43
   cancer 54
   examination 5, 38–40, 175
   infectious disease 51–3, 151
   obstructive disease 43–8
rheumatic fever 23–4
rheumatoid arthritis 102
rickets 95–6
rubella 147

sarcoidosis 95
scarlet fever 150
schizophrenia 142
scleroderma 104
seizures 131
sexually transmitted diseases 167
shingles 148–9

6 Fs 60
Sjogren's syndrome 103
skin infections 157–8
skin rashes 104, 155
    paediatric 147, 148, 150
skin tumours 156–7
small bowel 58
social history 5
splinter haemorrhages 16
squamous cell carcinoma 54, 156
statins 11, 15
steroid therapy 4, 46, 88
stomach 57–8, 151
stones, renal 109
streptococcal disease 23–4, 25, 150
subarachnoid haemorrhage 121
surgery
    clotting and 35, 117, 118
    in diabetics 73, 74
    respiratory disease and 44, 51
syncope (faint) 130
systemic lupus erythematosus (SLE) 104
systemic sclerosis 104

T_4 (thyroxine) 85, 86
temporal arteritis 103, 122
tension headache 122
testis 81
thrombolysis 14
thrombosis
    arterial 9–15, 75
    venous 35, 36
thyroid gland 85–7, 89

thyroid-stimulating hormone (TSH) 80,
    81, 85
transfusion 116
transplantation, liver 68
tricuspid valve 21, 22
trigeminal nerve 123, 126–7, 161
    neuralgia 122
trochlear nerve 123, 126
troponin 13
tuberculosis 53

ulcerative colitis 59
unconsciousness 130–2
unstable angina 10, 12
upper respiratory tract infections (URTIs)
    51
urinary tract infections 109
urticaria 155

vagus nerve 125, 127
varicella 148–9
vasculitis 103, 122
venous thrombosis 35, 36
ventricular failure 29–30
vestibulocochlear nerve 124, 127
Virchow's triad 35
vitamin B_{12} 115
vitamin D 95–6
vitamin K 63
von Willebrand's disease 117

warfarin 35, 37, 118
whooping cough 151

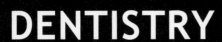
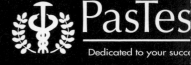